Transitions

Second Edition

Robert Milstid

1

Transitions

amazon.com/author/robertmilstid

https://rmilstid.wordpress.com/

https://twitter.com/robertmilstid

Introduction

3

Earl Hadley, an insightful and proficient handyman, takes a job with The Blue Lakes Memory Care Center; this choice endears him to the challenging world of dementia and Alzheimer's care, exposing him to the disease's devastating effects on the residents and their family members. Earl is challenged and pulled in myriad ways as he empathetically befriends the community's lively residents, all the while trying to overcome his own cathartic struggle to accept the reality of his father's suicide note that he has received fifteen years after the fact. His witness of the resident's plight at Blue Lakes could give him the needed acceptance of life's unpredictable journey, and allow him to become a vibrant presence in the last chapters of the resident's lives.

Contents

It starts with coffee

It's 5:30 am. My wife Ella brings us a tray with coffee into the bedroom; it is our morning ritual. We both agree that a day not started with a quiet cup of coffee is unthinkable and leads to crying. I relish this part of our day. We drink our coffee and plan slowly. Ella is clearly ready to burst with information as she snuggles back into our bed. I know her well enough to know that she has something big she wants to say, yet she is trying her best to honor our morning quiet time together. She can no longer contain herself and says, "Sweetie, look at this!" Ella shows me a help wanted ad that she has printed off the computer. It's a maintenance tech position for at a memory care facility. I smile at her and tell her that I think it looks a bit out of my comfort zone.

The job was a maintenance position for a memory care community. I had recently seen the Leonardo DiCaprio film called Shutter Island so that was the image that was fresh in my mind as I considered swallowing my pride and actually driving over to the building to drop off an application. My pride was getting to be very similar to the old bottle of truffle oil way in the back of the refrigerator. That thing that you always said you didn't want to throw out because it cost a lot and could be used to make a meal complete if the occasion arose. My handyman and custom carpentry business have been very slow since the economy took a nosedive and I've been contemplating taking on another job until things were better. Honestly, I wasn't quite ready to give up on my business, but the reality was setting in.

There was something on my mind this morning that I had not yet shared with Ella. I have recently been plagued with a new concern; a note that I received in the mail. It was from my stepbrother back in Texas. It was a large manila envelope with two letters enclosed. The two letters in the envelope were separate; one was marked to open and read first, the other one said on the upper left corner of the envelope, "Earl please read this when you can, Dad." The letter from my stepbrother said that he had held onto my dad's suicide note for the last fifteen years. He told me in his writings that he did not want me to be upset more than I already was at the time. Back when it all went down I was beside myself to say the very least. Everyone in my family knew I was upset because of how close my dad and I had always been. I had worked with my dad as his helper for years in his business. While growing up in Texas I started working for my dad when I was eight and continued working with him until I was twenty-seven years old. We repaired mobile homes and I was his maintenance man for approximately thirty mobile homes for many of those years. We spent time in the mornings together most every day when I was growing up; I had coffee with him most every morning from elementary school until the day I left for New York City at age twenty-seven to take on the world. I had always wanted to experience a big city and Manhattan had been on my radar for several years. I had a restless spirit and wanted to see more of the world while I was still young. It was so hard for my dad to accept that I wanted to move away, but to his credit, he was never negative about it. I know it bothered him but he put on a supportive face for my benefit. Despite his best efforts to show his support for my desire to seek out a new path, my dad was crushed by my decision to move so far away and give up my role the family business. To this day I often have felt that my absence was part of what drove him to do what he did.

When he killed himself, I went through a period of about eleven months in shock and was quite volatile. I was so mad at everything around me and I couldn't get close to anyone, including my wife at that time. I contemplated following my dad right into eternity myself at the time. I was so torn and even though my stepmother was a witness to what he did and told me about it, I could barely believe it. In time, knowing how radical my dad could be and the fact that I had heard him mention suicide on several occasions when I was growing up, eventually I did accept the fact that he did take his own life. During that time I did a lot of soul-searching; I was a broken man, my trust for anything and everything seemed to dwindle. In an attempt to gather up my strength, I worked harder than I had ever worked in my freelance carpentry jobs. I pushed my creativity in fabricating to its limit. Every new project was a chance to prove I was better than the pain that was seated deep inside. I also started to design a tattoo for my arm. I wanted a broken heart tattooed on my arm so I would never forget my dad; I'll never forget the night that I had it put on. After driving around for hours, I stopped in at a pub next door and had a beer before going to get the tattoo. I wanted to get it but I guess I needed help get my courage up because I had heard that the process was painful. I designed the broken heart on paper myself and brought it with me to have the tattoo artist transfer the image to my arm. I know how cliché a broken heart could be, but I wanted to hold on to the pain because in my mind it kept me close to the last days that he was still alive. No one around me seemed to understand that part, but I did.

After his death, I went through years having lost the desire to care what anyone else thought anyway. In time I slowly recovered and moved on with my life. That journey wasn't fast enough for a lot of the people around me but what can I say to that, it is what it is I guess. I'm so glad to have so many of those years behind me now. Perspective is a friend to time and clarity comes with age. The letter from my stepbrother went on to say that he was sorry for not sending it sooner but after a year had gone by he no longer thought it would serve me in any way. He said after all these years his wife came across it when they were getting ready to move. They both agreed I should have it and mailed it to me. I took my dad's letter and stared at it for about thirty minutes but could not get the gumption up to actually open it. I put it in the top drawer of my desk and decided to wait until I was in the frame of mind that could receive his words after so many years of wondering what had happened to him.

I've decided to sit on it for a while. Yes, I am very curious but I have a family to take care of and I lost a portion of my life already with the death of my dad. I don't want Ella and the kids to have to worry about it. I haven't even told Ella anything about receiving the letters; I don't want her to be worried. My dad's death was so very taxing on my first marriage. I have to give my first wife a lot of credit for putting up with me during that rough time. She really was good to me during that period of our life. We had more than our share of struggles as the years went on but that's a whole different story. I'm not about to let this tarnish my relationship with Ella or hurt her in any way. She doesn't deserve to have to carry this burden.

Other than a lack of work, our life is good and I want it to stay that way; I need to get back to collecting a check. No matter what is going on in my life the rest of the world is still spinning. That concept is refreshing. I know that this will pass and I will come to terms with how I will deal with the letter. After so many years have passed I have learned that bad energy is best left behind even when it comes to family. This will be my burden and I'm not going to put it on anyone else's shoulders, not this time. At forty-nine years old I cannot go backward, I have to keep going forward. I haven't had any work offers for over three weeks; with no big offers of employment on my plate and knowing that my kids were going to expect to eat more than once a week I decided to give the job that Ella told me about a shot.

The next morning I woke up with my usual two cups of coffee and eased into the process of getting my please hire me look. Ok, that's not true, I got dressed in a semi-professional but not desperate look and was filled with the attitude of "I'll apply and quickly hope they don't hire me." I was overqualified in my mindset and not committed to being a maintenance man again after so many years of doing it as a kid, teenager, and young man. I did need a steady job right now so I would be smart to keep my pride in my pocket for now, for today at least. It's not fair to my family for me to only make money and provide only when it feels good. What if all the birds in the world told their open-mouthed chirping babies that they just weren't feeling it and they would consider feeding them at a more fulfilling time? That's a random thought. I'm getting flooded with these thoughts this morning. What if they don't see me as qualified? What ifs are permeating my thoughts and that's not a recipe for success. I'm starting to get freaky about all of this. It's time to get a grip on my inner self and go into this place and get them to make me an offer. I'll just go in and see what they are looking for; after all, they're the ones who placed the help wanted ad online. That's good to remember.

I drive just past downtown and into the neighborhood where the building is located. I'm feeling a bit of anxiety over this though I'm not sure why. It feels important all of sudden to me yet it's just a job interview. I do well with this stuff. It's cool for a summer morning; I've got my windows down and Harry Connick, Jr. playing.

I'm wearing new khaki pants and one of my better dark blue shirts so at least I know I will look good. I can see myself landing a new steady job and going home like a conquering warrior fresh with a hard-earned victory as well as the promise of steady paychecks. Relax and breathe, I say to myself because it looks like I'm here. I take a right turn into the property. It's a large property surrounded by tall oak trees. They are very tall, old and stately. The landscaping is nice looking but doesn't have a pervasive slickness to it. I wondered to myself if overseeing the grounds upkeep would be part of job scope that I am applying for. Being a perfectionist at heart I already find myself making mental notes as to what the building could use. This is a better place to be in my own mind. They need help and I want a job. It's a win-win. While I'm pulling into one of the parking spaces with my van I see a really nice navy blue colored pickup truck pull in next to me. When I get out I notice that the man has parked in the spot very crooked. He got out of the truck and walked towards the main entrance of the larger building. Since we were heading to the same building I said hello. He asked me how I was doing and I said just fine. I decided to mess with him about his parking job. I looked over and asked him, "Park much?"

He looked back at his truck and smiled and said, "It doesn't look like it does it?"

I let him off the hook and told him that the parking spot had a weird angle to it, which was true. I introduced myself on the way in and he asked me if I was coming to visit one of the residents. I told him no and that I was here for a job interview. He wished me luck and asked me a little bit about my working background. I told him a couple examples of my recent work and we shared a little more conversation, then walked into the building and went our separate ways.

I would later find out that he was the head of our state's maintenance division. I must have made a good impression because I would find out later that he told the building's Executive Director that she should take a serious look at hiring me. That goes to show you that it's a small world and you never know who people are when you meet them for the first time.

I walked into the front entrance to the lobby and was quickly impressed. It had the look of a Victorian style two story home. The freshly painted white banister flowing from the second floor looked clean and well made; it complemented the raised panels on the wall that follow the stairs to the first floor. The curtains are all lush and perfectly matched to the furniture. It looks more like the inside of an old southern home than an assisted living facility. I walked over to the front office and saw the receptionist's name on the front of her desk, Sue, a smartly dressed Asian woman who greeted me with a warm and welcome smile.

"Good morning Sue, my name Earl Hadley; I'd like to get an application for your maintenance position."

"Absolutely," she says, "Thank you for coming in Mr. Hadley."

I replied, "You're welcome, I'm looking forward to hearing more about the position."

"It's a very important job," she said, "Let me get an application for you."

She smiled and reached in one of the folders on her desk and pulled out an application and brought me over to a private desk where I could fill everything out. She told me to let her know when I was finished with the application and she would then pass it along to the Executive Director, Mrs. Whitfield. She said if I had time I could do a quick meet and greet with her.

"Good luck," she said as she walked back to her desk.

"Thank you," I replied, as I sat down and filled everything out.

While working on the application several people walked in and out of the lobby area. Most of them were older and I assumed that they were some of the residents that lived in the community. About five minutes into my paperwork one of the waiters from the dining room came by and dropped off a cold bottle of water, I thought that was a nice touch. While filling out my paperwork I could hear all the day-to-day sounds of the office and its business unfolding; the phone seemed to ring incessantly and the kitchen staff scurried from one location to the next. They were serving breakfast in the dining room that was just around the corner. The oatmeal I had for breakfast was no match for the aroma of bacon flowing out of dining room. I had just finished filling out the application and looked up to see what I thought could be the Executive Director coming out of her office. She had on a very expensive looking champagne colored suit, and she carried herself well; she definitely looked in charge although her demeanor appeared to be pleasant.

She walked right up to me and politely greeted me, "Oh good, they brought you something to drink."

I stood up and greeted her with a handshake. She stood very tall in front of me; I had not realized how tall she was from afar.

She introduced herself as Mrs. Whitfield and said, "Thank you for coming in, are you here on the maintenance position?"

"Yes ma'am, are you still looking for someone?"

She said she was and that she would be interviewing several people over the next few days.

I let Mrs. Whitfield know that I was very interested in the position, I then introduced myself, "My name is Earl, Earl Hadley."

She replied, "It's very nice to meet you, Mr. Hadley, I'm so glad you are interested in working with us. Have you ever worked for an assisted living community?"

I told her that I had not, but the fact that I had over thirty years of handyman experience should make the transition to working in a community like Blue Lakes relatively easy. I let her know that I would be finishing up my application shortly and would be available for a quick chat if she had time. She said that she would be looking forward to reviewing my application, but she had a conference call that was going to be starting in about five minutes. I told her that was fine and to just give me a phone call once she got a chance if she was interested in setting up an interview.

She told me she definitely wanted to speak with me about the job and she then walked over to her office. Before shutting the door she turned back and said, "Thank you for coming in Mr. Hadley; I hope to speak with you soon."

I looked over the application one more time to make sure that I got everything filled in then turned it over to the receptionist and left the office. Part of me wanted to look around some, but I didn't want to get too attached in case it didn't work out. I did have a good feeling about the place. On my way here this morning it sounded like another typical handyman situation and I was less than excited. This place had some potential. I jumped in my van and hit the road. Time would tell if this would turn into anything. I let out a sigh of relief; job shopping can wear a person out.

I didn't hear back from Mrs. Whitfield for a few days and I had pretty much decided that she had gone with someone else until the phone rang late Tuesday evening. I was outside piddling with the everlasting, ongoing, never finished the process of cleaning my garage, my man cave. After years of special projects, supplies, materials, tools, etc., my garage is pretty much out of storage space and each new project that I wanted to get into required an hour long rearranging of my workspace. I turned down the U2 disc I had playing and walked out into the front yard to speak with Mrs. Whitfield. She sounded very energetic and happy to be calling me.

She asked me if I was still looking for work and I said that I was. She wanted to know more about me so we talked back and forth with each other for about fifteen minutes.

I told her that I was looking for a place that I could be of benefit. I shared my philosophy on how short life is and that if you're going to take the time to do something and be somewhere, then you should do it with gusto and with the intention of going the extra mile. I told her that I realized that might sound like a pitch just to get my foot in the door, but that it was true.

Mrs. Whitfield said, "I believe you, Mr. Hadley, you've got a great resume and we could use as much optimism as we can get around here. I would ask you to walk the talk and not just talk the walk. I get a lot of enthusiasm from our associates during their first few weeks then, not so much. That's not true for everyone, but unfortunately, it is for a lot of them."

I said to Mrs. Whitefield, "I think most people reveal themselves within the first couple of months on the job sites that I've been on. Everyone is on their game and saying what they think you want to hear in the beginning. I've run several crews on jobs over the years so I know a bit about what you're going through in filling positions. If you bring me on board I'll lead by example as best I can and I promise that I'll be the same man three months from now as I am today."

"I like the way you think. It's bigger picture thinking. Well, Mr. Hadley, I'm impressed. You seem to have a good grasp of what it takes to work in this environment and I think you will be a good fit for us here at Blue Lakes. I'm looking to build a team of associates that are committed to making the community a better place; it's harder than people might think as you were just saying. Unfortunately finding the right employees isn't the easiest thing to do. You have to have a certain temperament to work in assisted living. Working with the residents who have Alzheimer's can be really taxing I can tell you; if your heart is not in it then it usually doesn't work out long term. I can tell by your enthusiasm that you would be a great addition to our staff of managers. This position would require you to take on the management responsibilities for your department. I would also have to ask you to make yourself available for a manager on duty shift every four to six weeks. It would be a few hours on Saturday and Sunday for the MOD weekend shifts. Would that be a problem?"

I quickly spoke up and said, "If we're able to reach an agreement and I get to come on board, I would be glad to handle all the management duties necessary to run the department, I'm able to organize and prioritize very well. I would ask that you allow me some space to develop my approach to running the maintenance department. Once I get a good handle on what the community's needs are, then I can set up routines that keep things flowing."

"You seem to have a good heart Mr. Hadley and a good understanding of what we're looking for, I'm definitely not the micro-managing type of Executive Director. I have plenty of work on my own plate; I want someone in this position that can think ahead and handle anything that comes up. If you need me then you will have my undivided attention, other than that, I just need the inspections and routine paperwork to be kept up to date and the communities to run as smoothly as possible. I would love to have you consider working with us."

She then made me a pretty good offer. The rate was not as high as I had hoped but it wasn't bad.

She said, "I will still need you to meet with two other management departments to complete the interview requirements, but as far as I'm concerned you're in."

I wanted to take the job right then and there but wanted to think on it overnight; my dad used to say to me that good things are not done in a hurry. His advice in business has served me well over the years, so I've tried to keep it in practice. I told her that I would like to think about the rate they were offering for the job and that I would get back to her soon. She seemed surprised that I did not jump at her offer but then said she was looking forward to hearing from me. That night I decided that I better give this assisted living position a shot. What's the worst thing that could happen? I still had to make it through the next two interviews to get the job anyway so it wasn't a done deal yet. I called up Mrs. Whitfield the next day and scheduled the second and third interviews. They both flowed pretty well and it became clear that I was the kind of man they were seeking.

So they offered me the position. It was so great to finally get to this point in the process. I was really happy except for the fact that there would still be a multitude of steps to get to the actual first day of work. I was informed that my background check would still have to come in with a green light as Mrs. Whitfield put it. I'm good with that; I don't see any reason to have to worry about not coming up with a good record. There were a couple of speeding tickets on my record but the last one was over two years ago so I'm thinking that I will be ok. And there were a few more hoops to jump through after the background check. I would also have to get a series of Hepatitis shots as well as a Tetanus shot, and an annual flu shot. I hate shots; I remember being a young boy bawling my eyes out in the lobby of the doctor's office as my mom would take me to the doctor for school shots. I'm pretty sure I can manage this without the crying part, but I still hate shots.

Before I would be allowed to start working with the company I would also have to go through a series of training classes. These classes would cover all the relevant topics associated with what one might find in a memory care center. There was fire safety, blood, and air born contamination precaution classes. There was even a class on how to be an effective maintenance man. It took quite some time to get through all of these things but I respected the process. It made me feel like I was getting involved in something that was important.

So I became the maintenance technician for the Blue Lakes Memory and Life Care Center. My wife Ella was so proud of me and it looks like the kids will get food and clothing after all. All kidding aside this seems like a really good job. As I prepared for my first day I wasn't sure how it would all pan out but I was excited. I knew I would be able to handle the maintenance side of the job; the rest would just have to slowly work itself out. As I got dressed for my first day of work and walked out my front door of my house I had a bit of a skip in my step. I loaded up my screw guns, extension cords and all the basic tools that I wanted to have on hand for my first day. I'm up for this; I'm ready to take on the first day at work. I started up my van and pulled out of my driveway heading to Blue Lakes; I had no idea at the time the journey that this job would put me on.

A Germ-a-phobic's Nightmare

I thought my first day would be a quiet one. Most first days tend to be that way; you don't know what you're doing and you don't know where anything is. Mrs. Whitfield told me to ease into the day and get to know the building. She most likely knew that this being a memory care center would take some getting used to. I thought that I would be able to adjust to the atmosphere and I knew to expect to be slightly out of my comfort zone on the first day. Today will be ok I said to myself, no worries.

Well no, it wasn't ok. It was a bizarre day; the things I saw would take some getting used to for sure. I appreciated where I was and the fact that at least now I actually had a steady job, but the whole experience of seeing the people in their various conditions seemed a bit surreal. I am empathetic by nature, I always have been but there was no denying the fact that I had yet to be exposed to groups of people suffering from dementia. I watched the residents moving all around the building, there were some that were completely mobile with seemingly good conversational skills and then there were those that camped out in large recliners in the TV rooms. They were the ones that I expected to see and were probably the most comfortable with. My meager understanding of all of this led me to believe they were the content ones; I did not yet understand that they had only advanced in their dementia and would be up and about if they could.

Then there were those with walkers. I guess breakfast was getting ready to be served in the dining room because it was like morning rush hour traffic trying to navigate the hallways. I thought to myself, thank God they did not have horns installed on their walkers or it would have sounded like New York City in Times Square. Soon they all had their walkers parked and lined up all along the wall that faced the dining room. I was impressed that they were lining up so well. I looked at the wall and envisioned a wooden pole mounted with reins tethering the walkers like cowboys stopping in the local saloon for refreshment. I passed the dining room where the residents were having breakfast and find myself instantly the focus of about a hundred eyeballs.

I heard one of the ladies say to her table, "That's my cousin, he's staying here now."

I smiled and waved at her. The whole table waved back at me and told me they were glad I was here. Someone from another table said to the ladies that I did not live here I was because I was a schoolteacher here to teach her how to fix her car.

An older man called over to me, "Hey, come over here."

"Hello Sir, how are you?" I said.

"Son you know me I'm sure, but I just wanted you to know that I got here some time ago. I've pretty much lived in every place in here. I'm the master of the…" He appeared to have completely lost his train of thought so I helped him out and suggested that he was pretty much in charge of things. He seemed very relieved and said,

"I'm the master of this city; I built this damn place with my bare hands, most of it that is." I told him that it must have taken him quite a while to get it all built and that he did a really good job. I could see a calm self-satisfaction come across his face.

Feeling like I was ahead in the conversation, moving on seemed like a good move. I walked over to another table and said hello to a lady who was looking down at her food in what seemed to be a trance. Although I had yet to learn how to speak with our residents or even how to behave around them, I decided to relax and be natural. I was feeling a strange kindred spirit almost immediately with the residents; for most of my life, I have felt like I was just a bit south of what people expected me to be. I kneeled down on one knee and said good morning to the woman. She did not respond to me, she just stared at her plate. I took a second to see what she was having and it actually looked pretty good.

I said to her, "You've got bacon, scrambled eggs, and a biscuit. My favorite thing to do with a biscuit is to push my finger into the middle of it to make a small space in it, and then I like to fill it with syrup. Have you ever tried that?"

She continued to stare at her plate and did not respond to me at all. I gave her a minute more then started to get up from what I assumed was a non-conversation. I could see her trying to say something very quietly as I was getting up. I got back down again where she would know that I was still paying attention to her. She was saying something in a whisper that I could not quite decipher; I asked her if she could repeat what she was saying to me.

After about a minute she turned her head towards me, looked me right in the eyes and said very quietly, "When I was a young girl, I would do that with my biscuit." Her eyes opened fully and I could see a real enthusiasm in her face as she continued, "I enjoyed bacon more than anything in the whole world."

I was blown away by her response. She had understood exactly what I was saying. I don't know why, but I wasn't expecting that. That was awesome. I looked at her and told her that I agreed with her and thought bacon was one of the best things in the world as well.

"You and I are a lot alike," I said.

She responded in a low voice to me, "Is that what you think?"

I wasn't sure how to respond, I started to say something else to her but I wasn't sure where else to go with our conversation, so I told her that I would see her around and looked forward to speaking with her again.

"I hope so, you're a nice young man," she said, and then very slowly returned to the fixed gaze she had prior to our conversation. She continued to stare at her plate as I walked off.

That was interesting, I thought to myself. I enjoyed speaking with her but I guess I was caught off guard by the normality of our conversation. She seemed so lost when I saw her, at least that was my first impression of her, and I did not expect to have such coherent interaction. She was alive and intelligent in that frail shell of a woman, I would have to keep my mind more open to what was going on around me. It's obvious that I no idea what is going on in regards to the residents and they're dementia. I have a lot to learn.

As I passed through the dining area the bliss of my initial introductions with the residents began to fade. I was starting to notice another side of what was the morning dining experience, which was various combinations of drooling and cranky attitudes. I looked over at one table to see a fight on the verge of erupting over one lady's attempt to pour her orange juice in everyone else's coffee at her table. It was getting quite heated.

"I'll cut your damn head off if you don't leave this glass away from here!" shouted one of the men who was desperately trying to preserve the integrity of his morning coffee.

After a few seconds of protest from the rest of the table's occupants, one of the dining room associates came by and redirected what I thought surely was going to become a full-scale riot. I watched him calmly put the table back together and take the troublemaker back to her seat. Soon there was a quiet resolve that came over the table. The associate then redirected the mood of the lady who had caused the fuss by getting her to focus on how many food items were still on her plate. He asked her, "You must be very hungry, and did you get to try your eggs yet?"

She shouted at him, saying, "I have never had an egg; I just want a glass of coffee so I can eat everything in my plate!"

He smiled at her and asked her if she wanted more coffee or orange juice. Her whole demeanor changed once he started talking how good the juice was at Blue Lakes. He went on and on about it, I flashed back to the scene in the movie Forest Gump, where the man was going on and on about how the many varieties of shrimp were available. The associate went into great detail about the many kinds of drinks that were available at Blue Lakes, and after a few minutes of boasting about the varied drink selections, the woman became calm and acted as if there had not been any problems what so ever. The others at her table resumed eating their morning meal quietly, yet obviously perturbed. I looked over and saw a man at one of the other tables completely mesmerized by the list of drinks that had been professed. His mouth was open and he stared at the knowledgeable associate with fascination. I decided I better get to work; this was interesting but I'm sure there was something more important for me to be doing on my first day at work. Little did I know at the time that this was indeed the perfect introduction to the realities I would face while working at Blue Lakes.

I walked the building and began the process of getting to know where things were. There were many sights and sounds coming out of the resident's rooms that I wasn't sure how to take. The quiet bliss of the first day on the job was just coming back to me only to abruptly change into a state chaos. As I walked past a large room that had a sign on it that said, Shower Room, I was astonished to hear a loud fracas going on from the shower room; it was a woman screaming at the top of her lungs. There was actual screaming coming out of the room that sounded like someone was being murdered.

I heard someone from the other side of the door yell what sounded like, "Ahh! Help! You're killing my hair! You're killing my own hair, stop doing, and stay down!"

I was getting very uncomfortable with what I was hearing, it literally sounded like someone was in danger. There was a lady inside making unnatural sounds that I can honestly say it sounded like alien speak. I was getting very nervous and the feeling I should do something but I wasn't sure what it was that I should do. As I looked at the door pondering the thought of going in to save someone, it opened up.

A large black woman walked out and caught me completely off guard causing me to yell something out that I'm not sure was a real word. She smiled very calmly at me as if she has seen and heard every odd thing that there is to see from a person and said, "Oh, you must be the new maintenance man?"

"Yes ma'am," I said with as much optimism as I could muster; I was still a little freaked out by the screaming.

"Oh you are going to love it here; we need a good maintenance man."

I asked her if everything was ok, she laughed and said, "Yes, it's alright; Miss Baby hates to get her showers. She's fine." She then smiled at me and walked off grinning from ear to ear, and I thought to myself, "Miss Baby?"

Continuing on I was beginning to feel as though I was in a movie or something. I pictured Robert DeNiro in a white coat walking out of one of the resident's rooms in each hallway that I walked down. I thought at any moment the place would transform into a play by Marat de Sade. With these thoughts, I must be overreacting. This must be all in my head. This is not that bad. It's a dementia care facility, which is not a place that I have ever imagined myself working at, but it's a legitimate place to work. At least that's what I keep telling myself.

I should be grateful. I am grateful. I would be more grateful if I had not just rounded a corner of one of the larger hallways, only to witness a man squatting down going poop on the hallway carpet. I try not to stare. I flash back to one of the interviews where the regional maintenance director said that one of my responsibilities would be overseeing the carpets and floors restoration after incontinent accidents. Oh, my God. I continue on and try not to think about it. I will have to get back to that. It's not like I'm going to walk up to this older gentleman and say, "Hello, I noticed you're pooping all over the carpet."

No, I will be just moving along and try to find someone to tell about what's happening down the hall, then look for something that needs repairing. The search for work will not be too hard; it's not as if the community is shabby, just in need of some upgrade. The walls all could use some fresh paint and the grounds have very little detail. It looks like the vendors including landscaping have been getting paid with only a small amount if any, supervision. I'm going to up the ante a little bit right off the bat and set up some meetings with all of our vendors to find out what they see as their job scope. Once I know that I should be able to manage their performance. I'm still not sure about the long-term aspects of my decision to take this position, but as long as I'm here I will make positive contributions. I will just have to get into the soup for a while.

Organizing a building's upgrades using paints, plants, and carpentry is not much different than making a good spaghetti supper with garlic bread. You just get all the ingredients together and start marinating, mixing and cooking. I love seeing a project unfold. It's satisfying to see people's faces change from unimpressed to noticeable approval. I decided to start organizing the painting supplies I had seen in a storage unit down just down the hall. That would be a quick improvement.

On my way over to the storage area, I passed a family room full of residents. The activities lady was doing an exercise routine with them. I say with them, but it was mostly all her. There were two or three, maybe four out of the twenty or so actually participating. The lady didn't let that bother her or curb her enthusiasm. She danced and motivated the few who were involved. I stopped to watch, and a lot of the residents were checking me out. Some smiled, some looked curious; still, others stared at me as if they were looking at a face that had not seen in decades.

I saw the lady from the dining room earlier this morning that thinks I'm her cousin sitting up and participating. "Hey Donald!" she yells out at full volume.

I wave to her even though I'm not sure who Donald is. I decided I would watch and maybe even join in for a second more. I don't know why but I was feeling that strange kinship that I mentioned before. A few of the residents were trying their best to participate and keep up with the physical requests of the activities lady. I watched a man trying his best to keep time with the music by patting his hand on the side of his face. A woman sitting next to him tried to sing, but could not keep tempo with the music, but that was not going to detour her from giving a dedicated attempt. I watched a man sit back and smile as if he had the best secret a person could have. Another man in the back of the room stood up behind his walker and gave full hand and arm motions as if he were conducting the entire room in his very own production. Although there were only a few residents actually participating, I'm giving them all credit because it's a hard life and I'm looking at people who have been dealt a very difficult hand. I found myself feeling at ease when I thought I would feel uneasy. I was starting to let my guard down.

A lady reached out from her wheelchair and said something that sounded like, "Dance with me!"

I thought to myself, this party is on. I reached out and took her hand. We swayed back and forth with the music playing; we slow danced like a couple of kids lost in time. I was not sure how to actually waltz, but in order to entertain my dance partner who was obviously enjoying herself; I gave it everything I had given our limited space and physical abilities. I danced in front of her wheelchair and she did her best to dance too. I have not been blessed with the skills of a good dancer, that fact was not lost on the room, but the effort was there so forgiveness was flowing and my dedication was appreciated. There were a few ladies from the staff that walked up and enjoyed their new maintenance man dancing with the residents on his first day. They joined in with the dance and contributed to the activity with energetic hand clapping. An old woman next to us stared and smiled at me with excitement, you would have thought a bright blue light or something surrounded me; she was mesmerized.

The song came to an end and another one started. That song ended and I thought that this would be a good time to move along and get back to my prior mission. I noticed that my partner was holding on and not yet ready to call it a day. The music stopped and I looked at her and thanked her for dancing with me. She laughed out loud and she let go of my hand, releasing a yellow substance from both of our hands. I was in a bit of shock at first. I just stared at the goo that was connecting my dance partner and my hand together with a stream of falling ooze. I think I threw up in my mouth just a little as I tried to collect my composure. I stepped away and gave her a nervous smile. The yellow saliva or sinus drainage or whatever it was slowly broke off, freeing me from my dance partner.

The activities director looked over at me with a straight face and said, "That's gross."

I said almost in a whisper, "Yes, yes it is."

I walked off in shock as a pair of associates took care of my smiling dance partner. I went straight to the bathroom and washed my hands for about ten minutes. I walked past the dining area and saw three men sitting at one of the tables eating.

One of them called out to me as I passed by their table, "Hey are you going to eat?"

The food was spraying from his mouth as he spoke, and I tried my best to keep my composure as I kept walking. As I walked at a nervous pace I could feel a cold sweat building up across my forehead as well as a nauseous feeling in the pit of my stomach. I was becoming overwhelmed and full of anxieties. As time went on I was beginning to feel trapped as if I had been lowered down into a barrel of germs. The feelings were getting stronger by the second. I needed to get outside and get some air; this is what was racing through my mind as I tried to contain nausea. My hope was that no one would see me experiencing this germ-a-phobic panic attack. It was my first day. What if Mrs. Whitfield was to see me like this? I would probably be relieved of all my newly acquired duties and sent home to look for employment. I was starting to get a smell in my nose that was unidentifiable. It had been building since I started this morning only now it would not go away. I felt it filtering through my lungs and mouth and eyes. I guess it could be psychosomatic, but just knowing that wasn't making it go away. All I could keep seeing was images of the man that pooped in the hallway, images of the yellow goo flowing between my hand and that of my smiling dance partner's, and an odd fear was starting to bubble up inside of me. I was feeling like I needed a hot shower.

All of the sudden the building's germs and stains were starting to become crystal clear to me. The snot spots periodically permeating the carpet in random locations, the handprints littered with someone's breakfast on the private dining room's glass doors. Any other time I would not care if the doors were made of glass, wood, plastic or tuna fish. I was going into some kind of mini panic attack.

I walked over to the head nurse and pointed to the private dining room and asked her, "Why are there glass doors in a private room? That makes it not private!"

She looked at me a bit puzzled. I caught myself, realizing how ridiculous I must sound to her and I quickly walked out to the employee area in the back of the kitchen. I asked one of the ladies sitting in the break area where the back door was because I had forgotten. She stared at me as if she could not understand a word I was saying. An older Spanish woman looked up from her paper at the break table and pointed to the back hallway. I hurried towards the back door and looked at the fingerprints that littered the bar that I had to put my hands on to get out. I took a deep breath, pulled my shirt up to use as a glove, and pushed the bar to open the door.

The daylight was almost blinding as I pushed the door open. There was a lake a short walk out back behind the building. I hurried in its direction with zero caution for what could be an alligator-filled lake for all I knew. This part of the state is full of gators. I didn't care at that moment; I needed to get some fresh air. I needed to breathe the kind of air God made. I needed to get away from the smell and the yellow stuff. I needed to calm down. Once at the lake I took a few minutes to just breathe, quiet my thoughts, and look around. I knelt down and tried to relax; I stayed like that for about five minutes. Wow, that was quite a panic attack. I knew that I was a germ-a-phobe, but that was a bit of an overreaction. I took a few minutes to collect my composure and looked out across the lake as it occurred to me how beautiful it is around here. The fact that I was healthy and not having the kinds of problems that the residents are is humbling; I tried to focus on that. I had to get it together and put my man suit back on. This place is where life has me so who am I to be ungrateful? I took another few minutes and gazed out at the lake. It occurred to me that at my age I might be in a position to learn something from all of this. I began to feel better and I walked back to the building to go back inside.

As I walked back to my office, I noticed that everything was back to normal. I just freaked out in my head and no one seemed to notice. I guess when you're working with Alzheimer's and Dementia, my germ problems do not register so high on the Richter scale. I'm ok now and glad to be sitting in my office. I took a few deep breaths and realized that my office smells pretty good. That was a real panic attack; I don't remember ever having anything like that. It's over now and the time is passing quickly for the first day. I realized I would have to go slow and keep a healthy perspective. I could do this.

A few weeks came and went and I began to get into the swing of things here in dementia world. I've settled into a pace that allows me to stay on top of my work orders, yet I have discovered mountains of safety reports and equipment inspections that I have to do. The state has a world of requirements when it comes to safety inspections and regulations when it comes to the building's upkeep. Blue Lakes, to their credit, does a great job of building their own hedge around the requirements. They have rules to keep you from getting close to breaking the rules. It can be a bit daunting trying to keep up with all the paperwork and making sure that the reports are emailed to the corporate offices on a weekly basis, but I got a handle on it. If that is what they want to pay me to do then I will be happy to comply.

The thing about this job that caught me off guard is the interaction that my position would have with the community's residents. Handyman work requires a person to get from one location to the next. The thing about my new-found a steady job is that it's full of people. Not just other workers, but people who think they know you. There are people that don't remember that you just spoke with them a few minutes ago. The community is populated with people whom you've just met, who then swear that they knew you when you were growing up. Some boast loudly about what they see as the fact that actually, they changed a few of your diapers! These people may look just like aunts, uncles, grandmothers, dads, and neighbors, but there is more to it than that. These people have runny noses and they drool and they sometimes find themselves so happy to see me that they wanted to hug me and shake my hand…with odd liquids on them. It's not easy to maintain your composure when you're not used to someone wanting to give you a kiss when you can clearly see that they have just wiped something gross on their cheek.

This happened to be something that I experienced one morning, not one hour after I punched in. Richard is his name. Sir Richard the golfer; not being a golfer myself I have decided in my own mind that he would swing a club or two back in the day. This may or may not be the case but I have noticed he wears a lot of plaids and golf-type shirts so I think the label fits. Sir Richard is a very proper man. His demeanor is serious and his manners are the kind of manners that one can appreciate having around. He is courteous and always wants to give me a firm handshake when he sees me. I have given him the nickname, Sir Richard. He seems to like it when I call him this; his demeanor takes on a regal cadence when he hears me address him in this fashion. We both enjoy it. Sir

Richard is a good man. I suspect that I would have liked him in his younger years. He used to run his own shoe repair business from what one of the associates told me today. Running a business takes gumption and guts. Any man who puts himself out there in that manner has my vote.

That being said, if I had known this morning what I would be sharing with Sir Richard, I would have elected to pick a different work order to complete. This morning I stepped down from a ladder in one of the main corridors and Sir Richard was at the bottom waiting for me. I stepped off the last step, turned around and there he was, up close and personal in my personal space. He was so happy to see me then he reached out, called me by someone else's name and gave me the biggest hug I have had in decades. He then reached in, puckered up and kissed my cheek. He started crying and telling me how much he has missed me. He was obviously thinking I was his son by the things he was saying. I stood there mostly paralyzed. I liked Sir Richard and I know that this job is going to require me to occasionally step out of my comfort zone, but Sir Richard has just given me a bear hug and a big kiss on the cheek with poop all over his face. Yes, Sir Richard and I now are sharing what was only brown smeared poop on his face; now the odorous and unsanitary condition was on both our faces.

I may have mentioned earlier the fact that I have a small problem with germs. I don't know how I thought that this would not be an issue. I have always been the kind of guy that would wash my hands way too much. As a teenager, I would literally take three showers a day. I'm sure my parents thought it was a puberty thing and sometimes it was, but mostly I just couldn't stand the thought of someone's personal dirt going from them to me. I have to keep moving forward.

The day's end comes and I've since washed the morning's episode off of me. I have decided to let it go. This place is growing on me and residents like Sir Richard are not really a problem, but a blessing. I have joined the staff of associates that get this place. It takes a certain character to flourish and find productivity in an environment full of dementia. Some get it and some do not. The clock-watchers do not survive employment long term. I find comfort in that fact. If you are not happy where you are, then moving on does everyone a favor.

I suspect that I have had a bit of an extreme reaction to the environment here at Blue Lakes; I am truly grossed out by a lot of things that I find myself having to touch, feel and breathe. When I leave to go home in the afternoons, the smell still lingers in my nose on a pervasive level. I have asked Ella to change cleaning products at home because it's all I smell, it taints my food, even my clothes seem to have taken on a new scent. I have managed to get my appetite back lately so that's a good sign; I will adjust and adapt to Blue Lakes and all its idiosyncrasies in time. I am confident in that.

We are interviewing a new cleaning lady a couple of days from now. The one we had didn't have the dedication that a place like this has to have. I'm coming to see the janitorial position as paramount to a dementia care environment. It requires someone with a tolerant nature because of the constant spills and the incontinent conditions that our residents are plagued with. The lady being interviewed has just moved here from Texas. I see that as a big plus for her right off the bat, that's where I'm from.

Blue Lakes is starting to feel more like a calling than a job; it has an undeniable wealth of needs. It has needs that bring me a great deal of comfort when I see that my efforts make a difference; when I take the time to go the extra mile I have my own cup filled much more than I ever expected. My maintenance skills are having a positive effect on the building and things are already shaping up. My work order request book is up to date which will allow me to focus on actual upgrades. The signs out front that sport the community's name on it is falling apart. I'm planning on making a new one and that will give a better first impression as new and potential clients visit us.

That's one thing I'm coming to understand about this job, the families and the residents. The first impression is that this is all crazy, but it's not like that. We all have issues; we are all in the same boat and face struggles that are unique to us. We all just want something more out of this life before it's too late. Working at Blue Lakes and experiencing the things I have experienced here has helped shape me and bring an evolution to my awareness. I think I've been put here to meet a few people who have more problems than I do. I wonder if it's time to open the note up that lies deep in the top drawer of my desk at home. It's been fifteen years since my dad went away, you would think I could handle reading a note from him after all these years. When I see the family members coming in to visit their loved ones I can't help but feel they are in some ways, lucky. At least they get to say their goodbyes. I doubt they see it that way. They are in the midst of dealing with a terrible disease and I'm sure the forest is thicker than the trees at this point in the process for them. I hate that this is something they have to deal with. After the loss of my dad, I know what the separation can feel like.

For today I'm going to tuck the thoughts of my ordeal a bit deeper in my priorities; I don't really feel ready, maybe I will be in an open space soon. Experience has shown me that time is good medicine. I also know that procrastination is the devil's workshop. Working at Blue Lakes can be a germ–a–phobic's nightmare, but it's also a great daily reminder that life is short. The residents, even in their disease, are teaching me a lot about what really matters. Life is good but not always fair. As our days roll along and we get to the last chapters of our lives, it is comforting to know that there is a bigger picture than we might see. The face in the mirror is not all we have at the end of the day; we have our faith, families, a lifetime full of accomplishments, victories and if we're lucky, someone that loves us and is still healthy enough to stop by and say hello.

Lady Red Bird

She would call out the words, "Red bird." She said this time after time again. Miss Hattie was her name. Her old frail body sat in a wheelchair covered in a soft and worn handmade blanket. She wore colorful striped socks but no shoes. Her hair was white and her eyes were light blue. Her eyes were amazing. She had the most beautiful and piercing eyes I have ever seen. Maybe that sounds odd, but they seem to have kept their youth while the rest of her body is frail and aged. I never saw anyone visiting her so I wondered where all the colorful socks came from. The socks made me wonder if I should stockpile what I want to wear and use when I get super old myself. This place has made me think of things I never imagined I would think about.

Lady Red Bird would be basking in the daylight coming through the skylight windows of our atrium courtyard. That area was her favorite spot to exist. I say exist because to me her stage of life seemed to be just that, existing. I would watch her day after day in the atrium.

Her raspy voice would call out the two words, "Red Bird." She had a face that would go from a serious stare to a smile that would light up a room. She seemed to keep an eye on me as I walked to and from the hallways, and I smiled at her each time I passed by; she would always return the gesture. We had a growing unspoken friendship and I enjoyed knowing she wanted me around.

At least I assumed she did. I was getting that feeling from multiple residents as the weeks passed. They accepted me, and some were under the impression that they had known me my whole life. No harm was done there. If it brings them comfort then we all grew up together as far as I'm concerned. I was finding a good amount of comfort these days in my maintenance position. I've settled into a good pace that seems to be keeping my bosses happy. I do like it here, although the smells and sounds of my environment will still take some getting used to. I might never get used to it.

Today I found myself more focused on Lady Red Bird; a name I think well suits Miss Hattie. I keep her nickname to myself so as not to step on the toes of family members and visitors who might not get the connection. I mention family members but I have yet to see any visitors to Lady Red Bird. She does have some family I would think because of the photos I've seen in her room. In these photos, she is a young lady, perhaps in her late twenties or mid-thirties. She seems to be married or at least that is my assumption based on the man that she is seen with in two of the photographs on her bookcase. I believe there is also a sister from the striking resemblance of the other woman in an ornately framed eight by ten photo of two young ladies sitting on her nightstand. I have looked at her pictures many times while changing a light bulb, unstopping a toilet or during the weekly water temperatures checks in her room.

I admit that I do look at most of the photos in the rooms while I go in to take care of my maintenance responsibilities. I find them amazing. All these forgetful men and woman have had full lives and have gone to all the places that people go to. Many of them have had large and exciting lives. The bulk of them either came from or had parents that came from the Depression Era. This time was especially interesting to me; our country was in transition. People worked extra hard back then just to have food on their plates and shoes on their feet. World wars were fought and America was full of heroes. The pictures in the resident's rooms were of many different sizes and shapes, from foreign countries and cities and varied locations all across America and abroad. I love the black and white photos the best; I like them because they seem to be from a time when things were a bit slower. When I was very young we watched TV in black and white. I watched The Three Stooges, Lassie, and Leave it to Beaver. The dials of my TV would get me to one of four available channels as opposed to today's 132 million channel choices. Time seemed to move at a snail's pace back then; summer days were long and I would all but wear out the tires of my bicycle from riding it all day. Pictures follow us through time, giving us all benchmarks to say I was there or I did that. This is what the photos do for me.

There is something quite grounding in an old picture. It's the memories that you want to remember; they are the memories that we stole from time. They can remind us of parents, old friends or even youthful innocence. As time goes by so fast these days I take comfort in my own photos that Ella and I have out around our house.

I've got a great one of my dad years before he went away in front of some mountains in Wyoming smoking a cigarette and holding a can of beer. He was handsome and proud. Pictures are powerful. Most of the rooms would contain pictures of men in military uniforms. Men would get married in uniform more often than not in the era that these residents grew up in. With the wars that we were fighting as a nation, many would get married just before shipping out to their perspective stations or while on leave. It was good to be witness to the previous lives that our residents had lived. Their physical conditions and mentalities that I have been exposed to during their stay at our community is obviously not the whole story that is their lives. The strong friendships, family vacations and countless memories that are known by each resident are frozen in time and on display within the rooms. It is sad that they have fallen so far in their disease, but at least they were lucky enough to have had good lives and realized dreams early on. They had the benefit of growing up in the most freedom filled and prosperous country the world has ever known. They came from a generation that saw their glasses half full for the most part.

Lady Red Bird and her sister must have been very close. There is one black and white photograph on her dresser that shows them together at the beach. The two women were smiling at the camera with an excitement gleaming across their faces. You could see the waves crashing far off in the background as they appeared to be having a great day. I wondered if Lady Red Bird remembered this day at the beach. I wondered what she remembered if anything. I learned in one of my training classes that the people with Alzheimer's have a process that they go through that is a form of reconciliation; they are aware of what is happening to them on some level even towards the end so they try to tie up loose ends in their subconscious.

I wondered what she was reliving through her periodical proclamations of the words, "Red Bird."

Maybe Red Bird was a pet Mrs. Hattie once had. Maybe her husband called her that. Maybe it has nothing to do with anything that might be rational to the average person; it could represent something completely unrelated to the words in their practical sense. Whatever it is, it belongs to her and it's not up to me to take it from her with a guess.   She calls out Red Bird with a spark in her beautiful blue eyes. That's something that makes her special; we all need something that makes us special. I finish bolting up the tank to the toilet base that I'm working on; it will leak no more. That's a good thing. Nobody likes a leaky toilet.

A couple of halls down, I can hear the soft voice in the atrium calling out ...."Red Bird."

Uncle Albert

The man was in his seventies when I met him. He could still transfer from a certain location to his wheelchair, but as the weeks past, he would spend ninety percent of the time in the wheelchair. It seemed less humiliating than to have to remind him of the fact that he was losing his ability to walk. The days of endless physical therapy were finally coming to a close. He was forgetting how to walk; an unfortunate side effect of the disease he had found himself living with for many years now. The day he came into our community was pretty much like any other day. We had activities going; I was moving about taking care of work orders while the head nurse was directing the associates in their duties. A tall woman accompanied him on his transfer from Texas. She rolled him in the front door and into our community. It was unclear if the family had hired her to act as an escort or if she simply was a friend. She was dressed in a business suit and appeared to be very professional. She didn't stay very long.

I was proud to hear we were getting another Texan in our midst. We now have three Texans in our community counting the housekeeper, our brand new resident Mr. Albert Penderson, and myself. He had a farmer's look about him when he arrived. His jeans were new and dark blue the way they use to look back in the day before it became fashionable to buy worn out jeans from the mall stores. His short-sleeved plaid shirt was a bit loose on him and he wore slippers and white socks. His look was still strong in spite of his apparent physical ailments, but the one thing I will never forget is the calm look in his eyes. He looked all around the place, sizing up our community. He seemed tranquil and looked content. He wore a cowboy hat as well, soft felt and gray in color. It was getting to be fall so it would be common for a true Texan to switch to a felt hat as opposed to a straw one. In Texas, at least when I was young it was still common to wear cowboy hats. It is not a fashion statement; it is a staple of our heritage and a great way to keep the sun out of your face.

While his traveling companion was speaking with the head nurse and making the final transfer arrangements, Mr. Penderson looked over my direction. He watched as I was climbing down from the ladder that I had set up to change one of the atrium light bulbs. He then fixed his eyes on me and gave me the warmest smile I had seen in a long time. He pointed at me in a common 'how ya doing' kind of way. I responded with the same gesture, which would from that point on be part of our bond. Going forward, we would greet each other in this same fashion most every day.

You never know who will connect with you and who will not. Some of the residents swear that I played over at their house when I was a kid and some of them say I was the first boyfriend they ever had. My role changes daily here at Blue Lakes and that's a reality I've made peace with while coming to terms with my position here at our community. Most of the time I am just a maintenance man and sometimes I am an adaptable best friend when a resident needs to talk.

I walked over to greet him and he said with a strong firm voice, "How ya doin'?"

I made some small talk with him and started to go back to work. As I walked away he told me to go check on his room and to make sure that his things are put in the right places. I turned around to listen to what he was saying.

He then went on to say, "I'm glad they sent you in here early. I've been planning on getting over here to see how you were getting along but as you can see I've had a few setbacks."

"Things here are good," I said to Mr. Penderson, "I've got everything under control."

"Well that's good news; I was hoping you had things under control," he said to me in a slightly confused state, "Hell, I thought I did but then everything kind of went south."

After many varied types of conversations, I've learned to go with the flow when the residents tell me things. I've found in my experience here at Blue Lakes, that people can be stuck in different time periods or even stuck in a moment that they have struggled with at some point in their lives. I've come to this conclusion after so many conversations with the residents. I've learned not to get frustrated. Whatever they may be feeling or wanting to express is very important to them. Mr. Penderson was a unique old man and I could tell he would be someone who would have a strong effect on my time with this company. Mr. Penderson looks like my mom's brother and he reminds me of all the memories that I had as a kid that involved this particular uncle. Usually, the residents would look at me and see someone whom they thought they knew. Sometimes they think I'm one of their children, sometimes they see me as a parent. Today I've made a new and kindred connection with Mr. Penderson. It's a connection that I assume many of the residents experience when they are stimulated by a certain image or perhaps a certain song that reminds them of something from the past.

The way the residents react to the world around them might likely be based on a different memory, time or place that has little to do with what is literally in front of them. This may not be a constant effect but it is at least likely since the Alzheimer's does disrupt the signals that are wrapped up in chemical bursts that leave the stimulated nerves in the affected minds of those stricken with the disease.

We all have memories and life experiences that are not privy to those around us. People are complicated and unique. Dementia can go down a deep rabbit hole in its stages and directions. My revelation comes from the fact that Mr. Penderson looks like my uncle from Texas. I had several uncles growing up as a kid. My dad had eleven brothers. Mr. Penderson was the splitting image of my mom's brother. That was comforting to me especially since my uncle had passed away many years ago. I like Mr. Penderson; he makes me feel closer to my family back in Texas. I decided to befriend our new resident in the gray felt cowboy hat; I don't get close to all the residents, honestly, I can't. Some draw you in and the rest you try to give as much respect as you can and move along. It's just like in life, we're not close to everyone we meet, just the ones we have room for in our limited circles. Honestly, I think it would be too painful to get close to the residents because of the unpredictable physical ailments that Alzheimer's will inflict upon them. They can be doing fine and out of the blue, another stage will set in giving way to a downward spiral. In the short amount of time that I have been here, two residents have already passed. With the weight of my own thoughts concerning the afterlife, it can be a bit much. Still, something feels right about my being here. I want to benefit these residents and in doing so maybe I can reach a better understanding of their struggle as well as my own. I need answers to questions that I don't even know to ask. For now, I need to set these thoughts down and be where I am. That will be a great place to start.

I walked over to speak with Mr. Penderson and said, "Mr. Penderson, it's really good to have you here with us."

He said, "Son why are you being so formal with me? You know I prefer to be called Albert. Call me Albert like you always call me Albert."

I told him I would and that I was sorry about the name thing. I told him that I wasn't sure how he wanted to be addressed in front of the newer people here.

He said he started this place and everyone knew who he was, and went on to say, "Hell I knew most of these folks when they were just youngsters building these rooms and these offices here. You and I built most of this place ourselves, don't you remember?"

I shook my head in agreement and said, "Those were good times."

He said, "It was for some, not for others."

I had a pretty busy day ahead of me so I decided to move on and get to work, "Albert old buddy, I better get back to work and earn my keep."

He smiled at me and looked away as if he had lost interest in our discussion. I said I would see him around and he didn't even look up. Such an odd condition that can lure you in with great hope and interest then shut you out in seconds. That takes some getting used to. Still, I do find comfort in this man's arrival for reasons that go deep into my subconscious.

The days came and went over the next few weeks. Mr. Penderson and I have a bond that seems to be growing. I've made it a thing on Friday afternoons just before quitting time to get with him for a beer. I'm having a non-alcoholic beer of course since I'm still technically on the clock, but Mr. Penderson has a cold can of the real stuff. I called his son who lives on the other side of town and visits every so often if it would be ok to have a beer with him. He was good with it.

I got the idea from Mr. Penderson's first few days with us.

He would say, "Oh boy, I could use a shot of bourbon right about now."

Obviously bringing bourbon into a place like this is probably not a good idea; the next thing you know there'd be wild hooting and hollering and Lord knows what else. I think a cold beer will hit the spot and give Mr. Penderson a taste of the old days, times when he stood tall and didn't need to be pushed in a chair.

One of my goals here at the community to give our residents the respect and dignity they deserve. We struggle through our lives from youth to adulthood mostly seeking just that, respect. I've seen associates from time to time treating the residents like children and basically just going through the motions of caretaking. These associates usually don't last for one reason or another; sometimes it's because they don't end up having the professional work habits that our community demands or the larger than life hearts that it takes to walk a mile in our resident's shoes. It's not the kind of place just anyone can work at. That's ok; it's not for everyone but you'll never know until you try, I'm living proof of that. Mr. Pendergrass and I will be going out to the lake for our beer this afternoon since today is Friday. At lunchtime, I took a lawn chair from my van and placed it near the lake so we could sit together. I walk into the family room and noticed Mr. Penderson watching TV.

"Hey Albert, are you in the mood to get out of here for a bit?"

He looked over at me and said, "Hey, how you doin'?"

"I'm doing good Albert. I snagged us a couple of beers. I thought we would go get some air out at the lake for a little while."

He smiles like a cat that just ate a can of tuna fish, and said, "Oh boy, I'd like that."

I get our drinks and we're now on our way. Before leaving out the front door, I stop in front of the head nurse's office and ask her if she's ready to go have a case of beer with us?

Since I have asked her this multiple times, she is ready with her standard rebuttal, "I wouldn't be caught dead hanging out with you two down by the lake, everyone knows that both of you are nothing but trouble when you get together."

I tell her that we're going out to the lake to pick up girls.

"Get out of here," she says with a laugh. She hits the security code on the front door; we stroll out like a couple of real men. Mr. Penderson asks me if I've got some cold ones as he carries our beer in his lap.

"I put them in that cooler you're carrying; I forgot to tell you that I put them there."

"That's ok; I forget a thing or two sometimes, hell I don't even remember where we're going. Do you?"

I reassure him, "We're going out to the lake to get some fresh air. Does that sound like a good idea?"

He laughs and says, "Oh boy, I sure do."

To get more out of our trip, we take a longer path to the lake. Our time at the lake will be short lived once we get there because

I've noticed that he doesn't like to stay out for long periods of time so I prefer to go around the property on the sidewalks before we hit the lake. Mr. Penderson gets a chance to see the outside world and it's good to run into the occasional man or woman from the community across the street. They walk around our side of the property as well. I think the mingling reminds them that there's more to life than just the inside of the building walls. We get to the lake and set up our spot. Mr. Penderson counts on me to bring a mug to pour his beer into. The glass isn't cold but he doesn't mind.

"You ready for a cold one?" I asked him.

"You know it." He said with a grin.

I started to pour his beer into the glass and he stopped me with a request.

"I like my beer cold and straight out of the can if you don't mind."

I respond to him saying, "Of course not, I just brought the glasses in case you wanted one. I like mine out of a can as well."

If there's one thing I guess I've gotten used to is how our resident's minds can change at the drop of a hat. Last week he went on and on about how he only drank his beer out of a glass when he was a young man. No worries. I hand him his beer and raise a toast, to a peaceful evening with no worries.

He smiled and said, "I know that's right!"

We both laughed and drank our beers. The water is calm this afternoon; I see the occasional fish jump up out of the water. I'm thinking there might be bass as well. I keep my eyes open for alligators. I have never seen any out here, but I would never completely let my guard down. I hear about people's pets being eaten by gators. I recently heard on the news that a lady was attacked while swimming in a retention pond about twenty-five miles from here. There are some houses on the property across the lake. They seem to interest Mr. Penderson; he always seems to look over in that direction when we come here.

"Those are some nice houses over there," I say.

"Oh boy, they are really nice," he says while staring across the lake.

He told me that he used to live not too far from a lake when he was growing up.

Mr. Penderson took a drink of his beer and said, "The Lake by our house was a lot bigger than this one."

I asked him, "Did you have a boat?"

He said his dad always had one. They went fishing at least once a month and even more than that in the summertime.

I said to Mr. Penderson, "I love fishing, my dad and I fished in the Gulf of Mexico, and we had a small bay house that was right on the Gulf. It was in a small town called Anahuac, back in Texas."

"That sounds like some good fishing," he said, "I didn't get to go saltwater fishing when I was growing up."

I love that his mind is still strong enough to discern the difference between salt-water fishing and fresh water. The water is so calm in the lake; I take a rock and throw it out into the lake.

"Look at those ripples Albert!" I said with excitement.

Mr. Penderson then said to me, "Those are like relationships, son", he said. "You used to love to throw rocks when you were young. I still remember the time you broke the window in our house, do you remember that?"

"Oh yeah, how could I forget," I said smiling, "Sorry about that window."

He said, "Oh don't worry about that son. We decided to let that go."

"Ok, I think that's a good idea," I said to him realizing he was probably thinking back to an incident with his kids.

I'm just going with his stream of thought; I'm not going to ruin a good time with the facts. Not today, today was a good day and we were having a great time. After about fifteen minutes we finished our drinks and headed back. I wish I could spend an evening like this with my real uncle, I really miss him, but Mr. Penderson has blessed me with the next best thing. Working here at Blue Lakes is mutually beneficial, they get some good work from me and I get a building full of great friends.

One of the associates makes a comment when we come back in, "It's about time you two rascals get back home."

This is one the older associates. She is in her sixties and pretty much calls everyone rascal, it gets old but it could be worse. As I get Mr. Penderson parked in the living room I say to him, "Good night Albert, I'm getting ready to head out, I'll see you tomorrow ok?"

He gives me his standard goodbye saying, "Lord willing and the creek don't rise."

The Halloween Party

59

It has been close to five months since I started this job and I must admit I'm really enjoying it. The crazy smells and messes are now under control now. Our housekeeper turned out to be a rock star. She has this place shining like it never did before. The environment is much fresher and inviting, although I would not say that it was unclean before I came on board. I feel like I've brought some of the standards up a few notches. This evening will be the costume party of the century; or at least the most festive evening our community has seen in quite some time. The place is done up with plenty of decorations and holiday enhancements. Memories of trick or treating down the old neighborhoods of our youth are being brought to fruition by the sights and sounds within the Blue Lake's community.

It's Halloween and we are getting set up for a party tonight that I'm hoping will spark a few good memories for our residents and create a few smiles. I've booked a three-piece band with a bass player who will be playing a big standup bass. A man playing the standup base is not something you see as much these days so that was the first thing that got my attention when I first saw them. The singer also plays clarinet, which lends itself to the musical climate that we want to establish. Tonight the music of the 1930s will be the theme. The music of Artie Hall, Judy Garland, Tony Dorsey and other musical giants of that era will be played including my favorite,

Glen Miller. The band members go by the name Lightning. They are dressed in suits and can really keep a mood going.   I saw them performing locally a while back and took their card because I knew they would be someone I would want to recommend in the future. There will be a lot to do with plenty of people on the clock tonight taking care of the basics, but a lot of the staff will be showing up as volunteers. That is the best way to the have fun and freedom to really enjoy the night; it also demonstrates the dedication and heart for what we're doing here. I don't want to come across as if we are working in some kind of fantasyland workplace; as in any workplace, you can find clock-watchers and associates who are only here to collect a check. Actually, I have no problem with that as long as they do step up to the plate when they are on their shift. This community has proven itself to have much more dedication and associate dedication than any job sites I've been on; that's why what we're doing here tonight will be possible. I want tonight to be something to remember; as I look around this evening, we are well on our way to making that happen.

I watched the resident's faces and listened to their comments today and it is truly inspiring. The short-term memories may be out the window with some of our people, but their souls can be seen dancing within their smiles and uninhibited comments. Several of them today have watched the decorations going up and hooted and hollered with obvious approval. I think this is one of the holidays that will bring back youthful memories. This evening will be a good excuse to have a party and laugh out loud. It's not every day that someone gets to dress up in a costume; it's a good excuse to let your inner child come out to play and believe me, based on the enthusiasm of some of our associates, there will be plenty of eccentric costumes and characters to engage to look at. Ella and I call it people watching.

One of the resident's family members had a collection of different colored fabrics. They had run a fabric distribution business a few years ago and had a garage full of leftover supplies; they donated a bunch of shiny silver material to line the walls of the room where the band would be playing. They were one of the families that were able to stay close and visit often because they literally lived down the street. Most people's family members are not so lucky but most of them do their best to stay close.

There is an intense amount of pressure on couples as they try to take on the role of caretaker to family members who are going through memory loss and even worse Alzheimer's. Before making the decision to come to Blue Lakes they were forced to come to terms with the parent's loss of mental and physical functions. The emotional turmoil of seeing the disease unfold can wear on the strongest of relationships, all the while trying their best to keep up a household as well as their own marriages. Eventually, it gets to be too much of a strain. They love their family members as much as ever but cannot take care of them from either a lack of understanding of the disease or simply the lack of ability to keep their loved ones and the rest of their family safe and sound. Once they overcome the extreme financial commitments that go with dementia and Alzheimer's care, they can make the decision to transition to managed care. They are better off as a family having brought their loved ones to communities that specialize in this type of care. When they bring them here they will usually find the peace they need to carry on. Everyone's story is unique. Tonight is about letting go of those worries and having some fun. I wanted that for myself, the families and my wife Ella who will be helping out delivering drinks and food to the wheelchair bound residents. Working at Blue Lakes can be as taxing as any job, but all work and no play are not what we are about at Blue Lakes.

I was able to create a nice effect on the walls after mounting a few spotlights I had purchased for the party. The silver material reflected a nice blue glow because of the colored gels that I placed over the light's lenses. We had boxes of orange Halloween lights from the year before; enough to line the ceiling at the lobby entrance as well and several areas throughout the main rooms that we would be using tonight. I have three rooms fully decorated with lights and hanging ornaments and the chef had a dry ice machine that he uses at functions like this, which will make for a great special effect. It will be releasing small amounts of smoke throughout the night as we pass by the snack table eating and drinking the orange and green punch that he has custom made for us. The chef has made several substantial contributions to tonight's festivities. He has created a buffet with various foods in the dining area. There is an Italian section with bruschetta and plates of buffalo mozzarella and tomatoes, and there are mini calzones with varieties of meat and cheese stuffing. There is a Mexican food option as well complete with mini burritos and sopapillas. The chef also made a special buffet section dedicated to the residents who require special diets and food consistencies.

Two of the associates will be dressed as Frankenstein greeting the people at the front door and handing out small blue masks and goody bags. I thought the masks would be a good way to get everyone involved even if they didn't have a costume; they also added an odd effect seeing so many blue masked people mixed in with the crowd. The two doormen were also in charge of keeping our residents from wandering out the door. They are both tall so it made for a great effect for the arriving guests especially with the matching costumes. It was looking good in here, we've definitely gone the extra mile in setting the place up for the festivities; tonight will be unforgettable.

The guests were steadily arriving and it looked like every immediate family member and then some was going to be here tonight. One of the families brought their foreign exchange students that were here from Japan. They looked to be in their late teens. They were dressed in traditional Japanese Kimonos and both wore the blue masks handed out by the Frankenstein twins.

There was a family entering the building along with whom it turns out is Lady Red Bird's sister. Wow, what a treat; she looks exactly like her sister. In the picture, I wouldn't have thought they were twins but the way they have both aged, they looked like it. The sister's name was Mildred. She walked in with elegance, wearing her age beautifully. She and her family entered the building and immediately made a beeline for Lady Red Bird. It was such a beautiful image to see the two sisters seeing each other for perhaps the first time in many years. Their eyes were both slightly tearful yet full of obvious joy as they grew closer to the reunion. Mildred moved across the room focused on her sister, passing the masked partygoers with little if any acknowledgment. She held her mask by the elastic band at her side with one hand and held her other hand out in front of her as if she was parting the Red Sea. She looked like she was from another era entirely in her red sequined dress; in fact, she was from another era. She was at least seventy-five years old or somewhere near that. What was equally inspiring was the face of Lady Red Bird as she saw her sister coming her way. Tears ran down her cheek and I was able to finally get a more valid knowledge of the two words she has emoted since I started working here. She called out from the moment she saw her across the room, "Red Bird." She kept repeating the words over and over.

I walked over to the man that had come in with Miss Hattie's sister, Mildred. I said to him, "They seem so happy to see each other."

"They are," he said, "Hattie finally has her Red Bird."

"Why does she call her Red Bird?" I asked. He said since they were small, Hattie would call her sister Red Bird. Her sister Mildred's favorite color was always red when they were growing up, so Hattie gave her the nickname Red Bird. Finally, after all these months I find out that there is a real Lady Red Bird.

The man went on to share a lot of their family history; he said Hattie's husband had been killed in a car accident only two months after they were married. Hattie was able to purchase a small house in their neighborhood with the life insurance policy that her husband had left her. The two sisters were very close, almost inseparable, especially after the passing of Hattie's husband. When Mildred and her husband decided to move to be closer to their grandchildren, Hattie sold her house and went in with them in purchasing a new house not far from Blue Lakes a few years before Hattie had succumbed to Alzheimer's. After it became apparent that they could not care for Hattie on their own they brought her to Blue Lakes. Mildred had visited her sister most every day but then she fell and fractured her hip about a year ago and experienced a slow recovery. This was the reason for the delay in visitation. I was glad to see them together again, especially now that I had the inside scoop on her family's background.

The night was unfolding and the party energy was picking up early on. The tall lady who had accompanied Mr. Penderson on the day he arrived came into the party accompanied by two women dressed in black evening dresses. They received their masks and began to mingle with the other family members as their leading lady made her way over to Mr. Penderson. He was so glad to see her, greeting her with smiles and a kiss on the cheek. They spoke for a minute or two about things that appeared to be just small talk then she leaned over and whispered in his ear. He immediately stopped smiling and at once his countenance changed. He looked up to her and I think he mouthed the words, "That's alright."

That's what it looked like from where I was standing. The woman pushed his wheelchair over to the dining area to prepare a plate for Mr. Penderson. She pointed out the floating fog from the table's centerpiece to Mr. Penderson; his face slowly became festive and soon his mood seemed to be improved. I was glad to see him out and about tonight at the party; I think he is transitioning to another stage of his Alzheimer's. He is much less coherent and far less mobile lately. I wondered what the story was with the lady that came here tonight to see him; I'm not going to get involved, it's probably none of my business. I didn't need to know everything; I just needed to feel good that people were reuniting with their families and we were all getting a taste of something out of the norm.

I was startled for a second to hear Mr. Ernie Taylor coming from his room's hallway, blasting out the old Frank Sinatra song 'Fly Me to the Moon' just as loud as he could. He was living large tonight. His mood was noticeably different tonight; he tends to be one of the more quiet ones for the most part. Maybe something has stimulated him on another level tonight. Whatever it is, it was good to see him singing and interacting with his son. It would have been better for everyone if he had a few more of the lyrics under his belt. He only repeated fiver words, Fly Me to the Moon over and over and over. His son was pushing him in his wheelchair sporting a big smile. His countenance revealed a slight embarrassment but he was still pleased to be with his dad.

I asked his son, "Did you teach him that song?"

He laughed and said, "If I did I would have taught him more than one line."

The two of us laughed. The son and his singing dad moved out the door, to the outside patio. That was a good place to be as the night evolved. There was plenty of room for people to stretch out and get some air. I had recently installed outdoor speakers in the middle of the courtyard. We had Glenn Miller tunes coming out of them to maintain some continuity with the music of the night. The band members switched to some music by Artie Shaw and they sounded great; I was amazed at how authentic their music sounded. We set a dance area up in front of the stage. Right off the bat, several wheelchair confined residents were rolled out on the dance floor to get the rest of us warmed up. You could not help but bob your head or sway from side to side while watching these wheelchair dancers do their happy moves. They were so excited; they were time traveling back to the 1930s. You could see youth in their faces; the residents were noticeably relaxed and in a good space. The activities director had choreographed a few moves with them that morning, not that they necessarily remembered, but some of it came back to them as the dancing progressed. It wasn't important how much they remembered; what was important was that tonight was full of tricks, treats and music! Tonight would offer memory making opportunities for the families, as well as all of the worker bees here at Blue Lakes.

I looked around about an hour into the night to see many family members hugging and laughing with the residents. This is exactly what I had hoped to witness. It's wonderful. I love seeing the residents wearing the blue masks we handed out early in the night; they have big smiles and you can tell the excitement of the party is not being lost on them. I grab a serving tray from the kitchen and load it up with food and drinks so I can check out the front entrance to see how my twin doormen are doing. I'm sure they are ready for something to eat and drink. I was right about that; they unloaded the tray in seconds and were thankful.

I walked out to the front entrance to the building and saw a young woman talking to one of our residents. He was also wheelchair bound but full of spunk. He was almost always smiling every day, an exception to some of the others who have been here as long as he has. I walked up and said hello.

"He is in such a good mood tonight," the young woman said.

"I'm good good good good good, I'm," he stutters his words in excitement.

She interrupts him with nervous laughter and said, "You sure are, you're are good good good". Looking up at me she says, "My name is Belinda and this is my granddad; his name is Roy Pierce."

I said, "I know Mr. Pierce, we've had several conversations. Isn't that right, Sir?"

Mr. Pierce confirms our relationship, "I know this man. I know him every day. He is one of the good, good, good."

His granddaughter interrupts him saying, "Yes, I've heard about this man, granddad; he's the maintenance man. He's very good isn't he?"

I ask Belinda, "How did you know I was the maintenance, man? I don't think we've met."

"We brought my granddad here two years ago after my grandmother passed. He seems to be doing so well here. You've done so much around here; the place looks great."

"Thanks, Belinda," I start to introduce myself, but she interrupts me saying, "You're Earl the maintenance man, you're very popular around here. Several of the families have mentioned you during family nights. Thank you for taking such good care of my granddad's room, I noticed you were able to replace the glass in his medicine cabinet."

"You're very welcome, actually, I replaced the whole cabinet. I had a new one in storage, so I thought it would look a lot better. Your grandfather is awesome, did you grow up around him?"

"No, we used to visit him and my grandmother every year when I was young but we stopped at some point I'm not sure why it was a long time ago. When I met my husband we bought a house very close to where my grandparents lived so I was able to be involved in their lives again. That has been a blessing. My husband really loves him; he had a great relationship with my granddad. I wish he could have been here tonight, he would love it."

I told her, "I think I've seen your husband visiting your granddad, I've just never had a chance to meet him yet."

"That was probably him; he comes here and visits every once in a while, he had to go out of town this weekend on business but I've got my camera, I will be taking a lot of pictures."

"I notice a lot of cameras tonight," I said, "That's good, I had hoped to create some new memories here tonight. That was one of my goals."

"You really are more than just a maintenance man aren't you?"

I smiled at her, "No, I'm just a maintenance man. Thank you for coming tonight, it was great to meet you."

"You too, thank you for what you do here. We can't visit as often as we would like but it's so nice to know that there are people like you in my dad's life."

"Thank you, it's my pleasure. I look forward to meeting your husband too; ya'll have a good night."

I walk back into the party and notice Mr. Kelly, one of our residents, laughing out loud sitting right in front of the band as they played. He was having such a great time. There was a lady sitting in a chair next to him that seemed to be enjoying the moment with him. I walked over and said hello. She introduced herself and said that Mr. Kelly was her dad. She seemed slightly uneasy though, I couldn't quite tell why. I'm used seeing some of the family members acting nervous or irritated from time to time when they come in to visit; I don't think I can hold that against them. Having parents inflicted with Alzheimer's is devastating. I'm sure they are all doing the best they can. I told her to have fun with her dad and that she should get her dad something from the buffet.

"This is a really nice party, thank you for doing this. My dad is really enjoying himself. It was nice talking with you."

"Thank you, it was nice talking to you as well," I said to her, then told her dad, "Mr. Kelly you have to see the buffet they have set up over in the dining area. The food is really good; don't forget to check out the fog machine in the dining room. It's a great effect."

Mr. Kelly said, "You're a good man."

He then laughed out loud as I waved goodbye. I moved throughout the party and felt overwhelmed with the obvious success of the night.   There was a lot of laughing and the family members and those living here at Blue Lakes were creating plenty of memories. The dancing and festivities went on until close to midnight. The partygoers left slowly one by one and the atmosphere settled into a calm late night mood. I knew I would be staying a while longer to help with the cleanup. Mrs. Whitfield and several of the other associates were already hard at it. The night went by so fast; after taking out all the large trash bags that were almost bursting at the seams from the nights clean up, I sat down and just took a minute to look around.

Most of the residents have gone back to their rooms but a few were still in their wheelchairs fast asleep with the blue masks hanging off to the side of their chairs. I saw Sir Richard sitting with two other residents in the family room across the hall; they were asleep but he was watching TV. After a few minutes of rest, I walked over to the dining room and to pack up a calzone to bring back home. They looked really good. I kept myself so busy tonight that I forgot to stop and eat. I heard the food was quite tasty. I walked out to the courtyard and saw Ella and two other associates picking up cups and plates.

"Ella, are you about ready to go?" I asked. "It looks like we've got a few things left to clean up but it's almost all good."

She smiled at me and walked over and gave me a kiss and said, "Earl, tonight was amazing; did you have a good time?"

"I had a great time, thanks for all your help. You have really good hair tonight," I said.

Ella smiled and started to walk towards the exit door and said, "If you hurry and get me home, we can mess it up."

"I'm in!" I said with a knowing grin, "I'll meet you out at the car in a few minutes."

"Ok," Ella said to me with an equally knowing smile, 'Hurry!" She walks out the exit door.

This is good, tonight was a good thing. I looked up into the sky, past the stars and say quietly under my breath, "Thank you, God."

Teach me something

It's Monday afternoon and the new lady is due any minute. We are getting a new resident this afternoon that is quite famous; her name is Betty Bellows. Her arrival is a big event here for many reasons; one is that this new lady will bring our community up to ninety-nine percent full. With her and one more resident moving in we will have every room full. Compliments are flowing these days about how our building has turned into something special. Mrs. Whitfield has a good vision for the place and is steering the ship well; our management's team slogan is "The cure is not in the box."

Miss Bellows arrived at about 3:00 pm with her family. I must admit when she first came in I had to contain myself. She had a tall hat on that looked like something out of a Dr. Seuss book. Her hair was jet black and done up with elaborate Medusa-like braids; her whole demeanor was undeniably eccentric. The jewelry that she wore on her wrists were made up of multiple tiny bells that would leave faint sounds of ringing tones as she moved along. The crooked gloss white wooden cane that Miss Bellows used to walk with was a work of art as well. I heard that she taught elementary school for a few years before becoming famous with her artistic ventures. Once she began showing in the Galleries of So Ho in New York City, she was in high demand. When I heard she would be joining us at Blue Lakes I did some research to be more familiar with her art. She had a bizarre imagination; her work reminded me of Dali, at least on some levels. With her over the top personality, I was looking forward to having her here at Blue Lakes.

Miss Bellows had a reputation of accomplishment that exceeded her teaching elementary school although she insists in one of the interviews that I read that she firmly believed that was the pinnacle of her accomplishment in life. She was better known to the public for her artwork. She was not only a well-known painter whose work is currently still found in galleries around the country, but she has written a novel that has been quite controversial for many years about her relationship with one of our country's former Presidents. Apparently, she took a lot of heat for the things that were exposed in the book.

We rolled out the red carpet for Miss Bellows arrival. This was actually done for the arrival of all of our new residents for the past six months. We thought it was a great idea to have them arrive in style. I added my personal twist to Miss Bellows arrival by holding up a sign that had the words, "Welcome to Blue Lakes Miss Bellows" painted on it. I used an old piece of driftwood that I had in my garage to make the sign. When Miss Bellows walked with her cane it was like watching a slow motion action scene from a Hollywood movie. Her demeanor was eccentric and intoxicating to witness. Her head would slowly pan from side to side as she walked; her blurry eyes had the gaze of someone twice hung over from a many long nights of hard drinking. That being said, she did seem to have a sharp wit about her.

Watching her move down the red carpet was like witnessing an opening night awards ceremony with a Tim Burton theme. Her motor skills have diminished somewhat yet she had retained a flowing grace in her walk. Once she spotted me holding the sign she stopped in her tracks and just stared at me for a couple of minutes. I was starting to feel a little uneasy because her reaction to me was unclear. She then smiled and then laughed out loud asking me, "Did you make that sign young man?"

"Yes Ma'am, I made it for you."

"Oh?" She walked over to me slowly, all the while never taking her eyes off of me. Once she was standing right in front of me she said, "I like your sign, you're an artist young man. I'm going to teach you something."

She then she finished walking down the carpet and was escorted around the community by one of the ladies that had brought her in. I was so excited to have such an interesting woman in our midst; not that all of our residents were not equally special. I just thought she would help elevate the enthusiasm in our community with her background. Her staff that she employed came in ahead of her and painted her room with bright colors. She had her room completely redecorated to reflect her taste. They even hung two of her paintings; I got a chance to see them when they were doing the final stages of decoration in her room. I was amazed to see in the center of one of the paintings a small identical hat that she wore when entering our building earlier this afternoon. That was quite odd

I thought to myself. There was much more to this lady than her zany appearance.

The day came to an end and I went home. My wife Ella had made us some of her famous garlic mashed potatoes that I often lovingly called Marry Me Mash Potatoes. I told Ella how happy I was these days working at Blue Lakes. If she had not pushed me to go in and apply for the job I might never have gone. We are having a quiet evening together tonight; the kids are staying with my mom tonight so that is always a recipe for a good, good night.

Ella and I end the night as we do several times a week, with a game of chess. This is a game that fascinates both of us because of the multi-dimensional challenge that it provides; it is very much like life. You make a move and something happens as a result of that move. The more focused your moves are the more likely you are to achieve success. I personally tend to be overly spontaneous which leads to a less secure outcome. Ella tends to win most of our games of chess because of her carefully calculated decisions. I kid her that I am just being a gentleman and allow her to win, but we both know she is the better player.

As she puts my king into check and whispers, "Checkmate." I reach over and give her a kiss.

I'm lucky.

The next morning I showed up to work a little bit early; I had a hallway that I wanted to get some fresh paint on. After painting for about twenty minutes or so the head nurse came down the hall and gave me the news.

Betty Bellows had passed away during the night from heart failure.

Ella's Cape

When I got home from work this afternoon I was tired and felt very out of focus. Losing Betty Bellows caught me off guard. Counting her, three residents have passed since I started. I didn't anticipate going through this kind of thing when I took the maintenance position. The training classes that were given at the time I started talking about the volatile and unpredictable stages that Alzheimer's can bring on so I can't really say I wasn't warned, but that doesn't make it any easier to watch the residents and their families go through such turmoil.

I've backed off a little when it comes to getting close to the residents because their decline was so painful to be a part of. That being said I can't bring myself to be completely removed from it all; that would go against my very nature. I really like residents and I want to be able to be there for them in some fashion.

I've noticed Mr. Penderson is starting to fall into another stage in his Alzheimer's. He and I have grown closer in our friendship and it's like watching someone from my own family go through the disease. It is terrible. The helpless looks on the faces of some of the family members are much more apparent to me these days. I know that all of this is not my job, I was hired to take care of the building; and I know that the steady paychecks from Blue Lakes are a blessing to my family but what I don't know is how long I can keep this up. My wife Ella watched her grandmother go through the many stages of Alzheimer's when she was a kid. Her grandmother had early onset Alzheimer's and endured its effects for twenty years before passing. Ella doesn't talk much about it; I assume it was traumatic to watch your own family member lose memories and eventually the body's basic functions. My job at Blue Lakes seems to expose me to approximately forty-three people going through this very thing on a daily basis. It's like witnessing pain on steroids. It wasn't like that when I started. I like being a part of their lives. It's the note. The fact that I still have yet to open the damn thing is driving me crazy and the weight of this unfinished nightmare is getting the best of me. It's bringing back all the feelings I had when my dad died. When I heard Miss Bellows passed away suddenly in the night, all of my past anxieties rushed in to fill me up again. I thought I was over it. It's amazing that something so bad can retrigger itself back into your life as if it just happened. I know how to disperse the pain of losing my dad, I had years of practice, but I have to deal with this note and I have to deal with how I will go forward working at my job with the knowledge of everyone's pending circumstances. Maybe I should leave Blue Lakes. I don't know if it is healthy for me long term to be there. I could be overreacting to everything. I'm very confused. This afternoon has been taxing and I am so glad to be home.

The house is quiet this afternoon; I usually come home in the afternoons through the garage so I can get a glimpse of my man cave before actually greeting the family. My motorcycle sits all shiny and eager to hit the road. All my tools, my band saw, table saw, chop saw, winks at me as if to say, "Hey let's make some stuff." My electric guitar and amp sit quietly under a drop cloth patiently waiting for me to pop open a can of beer and to turn on the fun. Most days these things bring a smile to my face just before entering the house but today I'm feeling weighed down by Miss Bellow's passing. I'm quite taxed by the note that I have yet to read; I know I shouldn't do it, but I'm seriously considering giving a two weeks' notice and moving on to something else. Working in the world of Alzheimer's is not some happy go lucky occupation. The residents deserve my best if I am going to be there and I don't feel like I'm giving my best to them or the job, at least not lately.

I enter the house and hear the kids in their rooms watching TV. I go in and give them a hug and a kiss. They tell me three thousand things that happened at school while I sit on their beds soaking it all in.

"Where is your mom?" I say while picking up the stray socks off my son's bedroom floor.

"She's in the bathroom, I wouldn't go in there if I were you, I think she's pooping!" My boy says with a fully committed laugh.

"Thanks for the warning, I'll be very careful. I'm going to get cleaned up; I'll see you in a little while."

"Okie-Dokie Daddy," he says as he reaches out to give our secret handshake.

"Okie-Dokie boy," I reply while finishing our little ritual.

As I walk into my bedroom and shut the door behind me, I can hear Ella running her bath water. I grab the stool that sits by my bedroom door and brings it into our bathroom where Ella is having what looks like a very cozy warm bath.

"I was hoping that was you," Ella said with an inviting grin. "How was your day, baby?"

"It was good," I said though not in a very convincing manner.

"What's the matter?" Ella asks while sliding down in her bath water. She holds her foot up for me to rub.

I move my stool next to the bath and begin to massage her foot while unloading some of the clutter in my head. "I might not stay at Blue Lakes."

Ella said, "Why not? I thought you were enjoying it."

I told her that there was more to it and went on to say, "I got a letter in the mail a while back. My stepbrother mailed it to me; it was my dad's suicide note that he left to me fifteen years ago. I never knew there was a note."

Ella was shocked, but after a few seconds asked, "What did it say?"

I told her that I didn't know; I said, "I haven't even opened it yet."

She asked, "Why didn't you tell me, oh baby that must be such a shock after all these years. Is that why you want to quit Blue Lakes?"

I told her, "Ella I don't really know what it's about. Yeah, the note is really hard for me to stomach but it's just that everyone in that place is dying."

"You're just figuring that out. Baby it's a memory care center for Alzheimer's, of course, they are all moving on, but you've been instrumental in giving them some dignity along the way."

"I'm a maintenance man," I said.

She replied to me as she moved her foot out of my lap, "You're more than a maintenance man and you know it. These people love you. You're their family when their family is not around. I've heard you go on and on about your friend Albert and how great it was that he reminded you of being close to your uncle."

I stopped her and said, "He's dying! Do you know what it's like to watch someone you like die just a little bit every day?"

Ella responds in an angry tone, "Hell yeah I know what it's like, did you forget that I watched my grandmother go through Alzheimer's for the first half of my life?"

"I'm sorry Ella, I do know," I say as I stand up and scoot the stool away from the bathtub.

Ella gets out of the bath and wraps a towel around herself. She says to me, "Earl, it's the note. I know how bad it was for you when your dad died. I wasn't there, but from what you've told me it was completely terrible. It was fifteen years ago though baby. You have kids and a wife who adores you. Our life is good. We've been so happy since you've taken this job, I don't want you to quit. But if you have to then let's first find out what the real problem is because you and I both know that the problem is not Blue Lakes. It's the note or some feelings that are connected to it."

I walked over to the sink and washed my hands saying, "I know it's the note, of course, it's the note. It took me so long to get past all these feelings and now here I am, right back in the middle of it."

Ella followed me over to the sink and put her hands on my shoulders and started to rub my neck saying to me, "That's the good part baby; you're not in the middle of it all again. You've already done that. You've fought your way back out of all those years of missing your dad. You're an amazing dad now yourself. It's not ground zero; it's just an extra leftover detail to work through. It's just one thing. You're so much bigger than that. Let's do this together. You've got me to help you and we're great at working things out right?"

I turn around and say to Ella, "We are pretty good together."

She reaches over to me and kisses me. "We are amazing, you are amazing and I'm only wearing a towel so you should do something about that." Her towel drops to the floor. "Woops, my towel fell off," she says with obvious intentions.

I put her up on the countertop between our two vanity sinks and we start to make love I say to Ella, "I'm sorry about your grandmother, I didn't mean to…"

Ella stops me and whispers, "Shh, I'm busy." She smiles and kisses my neck.

I reach over and close the bathroom door and kiss her on the mouth and say, "The bathroom?"

Ella whispers in my ear, "Absolutely."

All of my thoughts of frustration faded to a passion for Ella for the next half hour. I'm so lucky to have her. I will work through all of this; I know that the note is going to be something that I can no longer ignore. Now that Ella knows about it I will just have to man up and open it. I will want to do it right though. I have to find a good time and an appropriate setting. I love my dad still to this day. I miss him so bad it feels like a knife is still stuck somewhere in me so deep that it may never come out. His decision was his and his alone no matter what the note says, I will find a good time to read it, and I still owe him that.

The Bus Driver

This morning I showed up to work a little earlier than usual. I thought it would be a good morning to walk the property and try the sprinklers out. I think we have some heads that are out of order. I've noticed certain areas on the perimeter of the property that have been looking yellow. I'm thinking that would be a lack of water, anyway, I want to run all of the zones and see which ones are working and which ones are not. When I pulled into the parking lot I noticed an older gentleman washing our community's bus. We just got a new bus about two weeks ago and I heard Mrs. Whitfield talking about interviewing new drivers. I guess she went ahead and hired one of the men she was looking at. I pulled in two parking spots away from where the man was working.

When I got out of my van I said to the man jokingly, "You can wash my van when you're done with the bus."

"Oh that would be my pleasure young man, just hold your breath and I'll be over in a few minutes to wash your car, but you have a van," he said with a big grin.

One of our associates, Belinda was sitting on the bench next to the bus parking space, "That's Earl Hadley, he's our maintenance man. Earl, this is our new resident, Hickey. His full name is Willy H. Williams, he likes to be called Hickey though. Hickey is a new resident with us; he says he was a bus driver for over thirty years.

His family says he loves to wash cars so Mrs. Whitefield told me we could let him wash our bus whenever he wanted to."

"That sounds like a good deal, I'm very pleased to meet you, sir," I walked over to him and shook his hand, "So you're the new bus driver?"

"You can call me Hickey, My name is also Willy; my name is also Williams. I like it when people call me Hickey," he said as he sprayed the soapsuds off the front tires of the bus.

I said to him, "Well Hickey I'm Earl, that's what I like to be called. You're a bus driving man?"

"Well I'm not sure just yet; we'll see how it all works out. I drove the bus at Yale University for years and years, they had a very nice bus. That's what I always say. I did want to get this thing shined up. You should never let dirt build up over time. It's very bad for the paint car. You know what I mean?"

I said to him, "I know what you mean."

"Mrs. Lady, your boss or boss, I don't know who she was, but she told me all about you. She said you were the best maintenance man she's ever seen."

I responded, "She exaggerates, but that was very nice of her Hickey."

"Oh I don't know about that process; I do know about buses though. I've driven for half of my life, already retired once but it didn't stick," he said with a childish grin and then he laughed out loud and said, "Sitting around will kill you."

I told him I agreed and that I couldn't stand to just sit around.

"Dirt can ruin a good paint job if it's not kept in check. That's what I always say. Life is like that as well Earl Maintenance; you can let something burn you up inside until you feel like a pressure cooker waiting for the whistle to blow. Like a teapot, wait a minute; I can't remember what the hell I was just going. Have you ever had something bothering you deep down inside, and it seems like the longer you hold on to it, the harder it is to get free from it? I can't keep these things washed in. Wait a minute! I washed in. Oh hell, I lost my words. You know what I mean, don't you?"

"I think I do Hickey," I was taken aback by the old man's insightful thoughts. Even in his broken stream of thought, I could tell what he meant, at least I assumed that I could. After a few seconds said, "It's funny you would ask that. Lately, I've had a dose of that very thing."

The old man said, "I could tell that about you. After sixty-six years of living, it gets easier to see people and their mind words. That's what I always say. We've all had our ups and downs son. Look around at this place of the cars. Wait a minute; I forgot what you call the things. Cars and trucks are on the road."

"You mean parking lot?" I say trying to feed him just enough to help him out.

"That's the dang think, it's a parking lot; you know how I know it's a parking lot?" He says with a grin.

"How do you know," I asked curiously.

"Because it's filled with struggle, parking lots are filled with struggle. That's what I always say. I like that van you pulled up in. If you keep that van washed, the struggle will look great and you will get to enjoy it knowing you've done all you can do to keep the paint job clean and fresh. Wait a minute, yes now the transmission and the oil and the spark plugs, those are on the inside but much more important to the life of a vehicle. Those cars and bus things bothering you need to be flushed out and replaced with something good. That will keep your motor running smooth and will what you want to have happened, magically happen. That's what I always say."

"Hickey that's pretty deep stuff for this early in the morning," I said with a smile. "I better get to work, you have a good day Hickey. It was good to talk with you, let's talk again real soon."

He stepped back to dip his washcloth back in the soapy water and said something in a low voice. I could not understand what he said, I started to ask again but one of the associates drove by with her music playing very loud. She was singing out loud as if she was in the shower. I waved at her as she drove by and then turned back to the old man and said, "Sorry about that, I didn't catch what you were saying?" When I looked back to finish our conversation he was walking towards the front entrance to the community.

"He tends to walk off in mid-conversation; I'm surprised he talked with you as long as he did," Belinda said. "I'll see you later Earl, I have to catch up to Hickey."

"Ok," I said, I'll see ya'll inside in a little while. You better run," I told her with a kidding smile.

She responded, "I know that's right."

What an odd conversation. I have to say; I'm thinking the new resident Hickey and I are going to have some good talks. I decided to go get punched in so I could get on the sprinkler system. I finished out the morning and found several broken sprinkler heads. That would be easy to fix, I assume the lawn service may have hit them when they were mowing the lawn. The last time they were here I saw them repairing one that they had hit. They are pretty honest about that stuff and I appreciate it. They do really good work these days since they have realized that someone was holding them accountable. Sometimes that's all it takes, at least that's what I found in my dealings with the many vendors that we use in our community. About mid-day I went into Mrs. Whitfield's office to let her know that I was going to go out to purchase some parts to repair our sprinkler system. I asked her if she needed anything while I was out.

"We need a bench to go on the back side of the property. Actually, if they have something that looks good, get a couple. I want to set them out by the lake where you and Mr. Penderson have your man time."

"Man time?" I said with a grin.

She laughed and said she was very appreciative of the time I have been giving to the residents, "They need the interaction. I think it helps them to feel more at home. You're doing a great job Earl; we are lucky to have you."

"Thanks, oh, by the way, I met your new bus driver," I said as I started to walk out of her office.

"He's a very interesting man. He reminds me of you, only slightly older," she says with a mischievous laugh. "He is a very deep thinker, at least he was. He tells everyone that he was a retired bus driver, but his family says that he was a psychology professor at Yale. None of his family seems to know why he is so adamant about the bus driver thing."

"So you think he's like me?" I say.

She says, "Just the deep thinking part."

I tell Mrs. Whitfield, "I'm just a guy with a bag of tools."

"Yeah right and I'm just a bus driver," she says, "I'll see you later Earl."

I walked out of her office and out into the parking lot and looked over where we keep out new bus parked. It looks clean and shiny. Even though he gets lost in his words, Hickey was very insightful. He will be good for the community. Every day is something new here at Blue Lakes; I like that.

Warrior Children

A world of war is breaking out; the neuron forest plays host to the battleground filled with memories, feelings, and thoughts. The microscopic chemical bursts born from their mother nerve do battle with the highly disruptive Alzheimer's disease; this non-fictitious memory war wages on to this very day on multiple levels in The United States of America as well as the rest of the world. If I were a better man I would invent ways to heal the broken spirits of another set of victims of the Alzheimer's disease, the children.

When the front doorbell at Blue Lakes Memory and Life Care Center rings it is either a delivery or a family member for the most part. When I first started working here I didn't see answering the door as part of my job description. One of the things that life has taught me this past year is that "It's not my job," is just about the worst kind of thinking a person can have while on the clock or anywhere else you might find yourself. It leads to apathy and kills ones' potential for discovery. I now race to the door as it rings because I have come to realize that that few seconds of time spent by the visitor waiting for someone to answer the door can be a lifetime. It can be a peaceful transition from the outside world's burdens or a vehement supply of hostile anticipations. The children of Alzheimer's are forced into the caretaking role; I say forced because unless you deliberately go into the medical field with the physician's oath firmly placed under your arm, then you are receiving this job description against your will. It can be a prison sentence in many ways. You can look out your small window and dream of a time when things were different; you can curl up and think warm thoughts even though you know that the monstrous disease warden has fixed the thermostat's temperature so cold to keep you feeling helpless and in a congealed state. It is the disease that first kills the caretaker because the love of a child is hopeful and enduring and since the cure is still unrealized, hope will remain a thorn in the children of Alzheimer's victim's side.

Acceptance is a good place to start the healing process. While working at Blue Lakes, I see the transition of acceptance in the seasoned children. Once they have been able to relinquish the frustration of not being able to fix their loved ones and are able to receive the help they need, a calm will be evident in their stride. I notice that when the married couples first come to Blue Lakes to bring their loved ones they come in pairs, at least most of the time they do. I would say seventy-five percent of the time the child of the parent staying with us tends to be the more frequent visitor after the initial drop off. I don't know if that is a reflection on their marriages or just the realities of work schedules within their families. This disease can pull a person left and right and down at the drop of a hat. Releasing the burdens of guilt is a good place to start in the search for a peaceful end to this world war that is being fought by children of Alzheimer's. It's not your fault is good medicine; a mental picnic when you are away and taking care of the rest of your family is good medicine.

One day on the way into my office a resident walked up to me and said, "Are you the doctor?"

I said to her, "No ma'am, I'm just the maintenance man. I take care of the building to make sure it is safe and working properly."

"Oh ok. Well you look like a doctor, are you sure you're not able to get me my medicine, it will only take sixteen minutes," she said with anticipation.

"I wish I was a doctor. If I were I would definitely help you. I think the doctor will be in soon so you don't need to worry," I told her. After finishing up a report in my office, I came back out approximately fifteen minutes later.

The woman came up to me with the same nervous anticipation and said, "Are you the doctor?"

I know when a parent forgets the identity of their children, it is a deep and painful penetrating bruise on their children's psyche. The only way to find peace in your mom or dad's forgetful state is to accept that it is not their fault and definitely not personal. They still love you like they used to. They simply can't remember certain portions of their lives within any given set of moments. What we can't see is all of the times they may remember how much they desperately love you and miss you. It could happen early in the mornings or late at night. It may be less apparent once the disease is in high gear, but I personally think the mind is constantly searching for its way back to sanity. The chemical bursts from nerve stimulation will be misdirected and rerouted to an unnatural path while it looks for the correct destination. The body naturally wants to do the right thing so occasionally it could and most likely do get a clear signal to its correct destination, and consequently, a parent gets to relive an established memory and relationship.

Children of Alzheimer's are warriors; they battle and fight their way to acceptance. Some come out with the sanity of coming to grips with their parent's or friend's disease; some carry the burdens and the guilt of helplessness within themselves for years after their loved ones passing. We are all doing the best we can with the level of cognizance we are blessed with as we grow and move through this winding road that is our lives. At some point in time, there will be cures discovered that will disarm the Alzheimer's disease. Until that wonderful day comes, take up your battle swords and armor all you warrior children. Don't forget to count the blessings you still have. Life is good and bad and we are rich in spirit. As we take our battle rams and pound the doors of dementia, take heart. Soon we will storm the castle that holds the key to the cure. We move forward, and we continue to love our family. We win in the end one way or another. Stay strong until that day comes. You are worthy. You are warriors.

The Five-Minute Blessing

Time is moving along at a steady pace. I've decided to spend the next few days with a new focus on my job and the residents that I am blessed to know at Blue Lakes. I will get to the note one day soon but I feel the need to simply let it go for a few days. The clutter is not helping me go forward and I want nothing more than to get back to the clarity that this job has offered me in spite of receiving the two letters. The experience of running the maintenance department and interacting with the residents within the Blue Lakes community has taught me the value of time. Priorities will dictate your path. It only takes a minute to change your whole life. You can get a call that says you've got the new job you have been interviewing for or a phone call that lets you know your dog was hit by a car. I've learned to at least try to find the value of a minute with the residents, associates, my bosses and the family members here at Blue Lakes. In this day and age, everyone seems to be obsessed with multi-tasking, looking at his or her e-mail, tweeting, blogging, texting, or trying to keep up with whatever the newest technology is. I'm guilty of this as well but lately, I've developed a new habit. I've been attempting to learn how to make time stand still. Time is only the minutes ticking away on a clock that we have giving tremendous power. I think you can make time much less powerful in a conscience effort to gently take back the urgency that we have given it. If you think about the best times of our lives were when we found ourselves living and enjoying being exactly where we were when that special moment was taking place. We weren't staring at our watches.

This new experiment I've been working on is called the five-minute blessing. It is multi-dimensional in its concept and execution; for example, with the simple choice of giving someone the gift of full attention, you can literally change their state as well as your own. The simple choice of actually listening to someone and hearing him or her can be a ground-rattling experience. It's harder to do these days than people think. It's becoming a lost art. Think about how powerful a good piece of theater can be or even a movie. You still your mind and listen; you are transformed into a receptive state and it can be magical. If you were to take that same focus in an interaction with a real person, absent of wondering how much you still need to get done and focused on hearing someone tell you what they are feeling, and you will bless them. I personally believe that all of the great blessings in our world can be traced back to God; that's just my opinion, not the gospel. We are vessels in the blessing process if we chose to be. If I could bottle this concept I'm sure there are marriages that would flourish and customers that would always come back. The simple yet nearly impossible task of being where you are and actually in the moment can be miracles incarnate.

No one expects to be listened to these days. People say "How ya doing?" but they don't really want to know. If I ask my wife how her day was because I do want to know the high points, the quick main points of what she did in her day but I don't really want the book. I want the cliff notes. I suspect that's what she wants from me when she asks as well. Everyone can be affected by a few minutes of pure attention. It's a rarity and if you try it the results will always be good if you do it without wanting something in return. It can't fail. If you give five minutes of unbridled attention to someone without feeling the need to counter everything being said with what you really want to say, you will change the dynamic of the relationship with the person you are interacting with tenfold.

When I'm going from one work order to the next I try to keep my antenna up for who is doing what in the community. It is a practice that management here at Blue Lakes has been pushing and for good reason. Some of the residents who are several stages deep in their Alzheimer's tend to go into an introverted state. Some of them will keep their eyes involved with the surroundings while others, not so much. Their state of mind is the result of the level of dementia or Alzheimer's they are experiencing; other than that they are just like us in their desire to interact and have a good day. At least once a day I try to stop by to visit with someone and give the five- minute blessing. What I really like about my job here is that I get to fix things and make things but the powers that be within this company have asked employees to actually take time and show compassion to the residents that stay with us. That is very cool. I'm getting paid to help people feel good. That is part of the five-minute blessing as well; I'm not saying that other people haven't already tried variations that are just as good if not better, but this is what has worked for me.

Working here has helped me to see and relate to people a bit differently. When you take the focus off of yourself you tend to learn a lot. People tend to be quite self-absorbed, I know I am at least most of the time I am. When you're talking you're not learning. My five-minute blessing is an experiment in getting all of my attention and energy focused on someone other than myself. It does no good to stand over someone in a wheelchair and emote great words of empathy if you are not honestly being empathetic. The truth is powerful and it can set you free in any environment. If you don't know what to say then say that. Simple honesty will get a conversation or interaction off to a good start every time. It's easy to tell when someone is just going through the motions in a conversation. In our hurried lives, unfortunately, it can be the norm.

Relating to someone with dementia requires a willingness to step out of one's comfort zone and to suspend your own personal reality. If you are willing to step into the perceived reality of someone stricken with dementia then you have a good chance at making a connection. If they are staring at a door and insisting that they used to live on the other side, and then why not ask, "Was it a good place to live?" That's joining their reality and is also part of the five- minute blessing. That simple connection of exchanging two or three sentences that were mutually understood could be a powerful gift, especially to someone who doesn't feel that anyone is able to understand them anymore. A full few minutes of focused time together can make your week. Being in the moment takes patience and a decision to be where you are at that very minute with the one you want to speak with. Notice I said to speak with instead of speak to. The key is to get the focus off of yourself; stop trying to be heard and just listen. Give the other person the blessing of your full attention.

I practice on my wife without her knowing sometimes. That might sound tricky but if she gets to be heard and has all of my attention from time to time then I doubt she cares why I'm doing it. It's a win-win. She then treats me like a king and I get to see her in a blissful state for a while. If I were smart I would practice that behavior on a more consistent level, but I've got this whole only human thing going on. You've got to take the joy when you can get it.

I've learned so much. I feel like God has and is using me as a vehicle of some sort. I mean that in the humble sense. I'm just a handyman with a bag of tools; I think God uses everyone that will let him. To connect fully with the residents I've found another very important tool and that is to get down on one knee and get in front of them and look them in the eye. That sounds elementary but it is sometimes imperative, especially when someone is in a wheelchair. If they can't see your face then they probably won't want to engage in a meaningful interaction. You have to be willing to get into the soup as it were. The connection will most easily come from each of you while making eye contact. That is always the starting point. Once eye contact is made the bigger blessing begins. When I come across a resident that has his or her eyes shut and I'm sure they are actually awake I will reach out and touch them. Touching and exchanging energy is powerful; you can simply touch someone on the shoulder and pretty much change their physical state. Most of the people in my community have some form of dementia. Once they have gotten to this point they usually are not getting the physical interaction with people that we all need. How would you like to go long bouts of time without a meaningful touch? It is in our being to want and require touch. When I'm walking through the building I look around at our residents and wonder how long has it been since this person has been acknowledged for whom he is as opposed to what he needs? When have they been touched or even hugged? I can't imagine going days or weeks without being hugged. That sounds stinky.

Today I stopped and spoke with a man who tends to just stare straight forward. He will say a few words here and there but it is always in a low voice that can barely be heard. Daddy Bear is what people call him. I don't know why he has that name. He does have family members come in on the weekends from what I hear. I generally don't work weekends so I have always been away when they stopped by to visit. I hear that they call him Daddy Bear so that works for me. When I stopped to speak with him this morning I could tell he had been crying. He was staring forward as usual, and his eyes were red from having been crying so I asked him what was going on. After about a minute of waiting for his reply, I kneeled down in front of him and gave him a smile. I wanted to help him not to feel embarrassed about his state after all a man really doesn't want another man to see him crying. I said, "Hey Mr. Bear, were you able to get some breakfast this morning?"

He didn't respond, so I continued, "I saw that they were serving pancakes but I didn't see if you had a chance to get any."

He then said, "I got some, they were good."

"That's good," I said, "What's going on now, I noticed you looked kind of sad."

He stared straight ahead for a minute then he looked right at me and said, "I miss my daughter!"

I took my time in answering him because I wanted him to know that I had heard him.

"I'm sorry you're feeling sad, she must be a really great daughter," I said. After about a minute of waiting to see if he had anything else to say I broke the silence and told him that I had a daughter too and that he and I are in the same boat because I miss my daughter as well. I asked him how long it has been since they last spoke; he didn't seem to know. I told him that I would make an effort to see how she was and would get back to him with some information as soon as I could. I told him that it's ok to miss her and that that's normal.

He looked at me again and said, "That is normal."

"Of course it is," I said with a smile. I gave him a light guy slap on the arm and told him that I enjoyed speaking with him. He thanked me and I moved on down the hall and went back to work.

The five-minute blessings are sometimes powerful and sometimes are not much more than a quick, honest conversation. You never know what you'll get until you're there and experience it. Even if nothing big happens, you've given yourself and someone else five minutes of time spent in good old fashion technology free human interaction. Sometimes when you really set out to bless someone what ends up happening is that you are the one who gets truly blessed. It's like the old saying; the only thing you get to keep in this life is what you are willing to give away.

The Beach

I've taken a few days off from work. My paid time off was starting to really accumulate because I have a tendency not to use it. I don't have to work weekends except for every six weeks or so as Manager on Duty so that usually fills my cup. Baseball season is on its way out. My son only has one more game for the season so I'm going to take some time to work out the things that have been on my mind. I feel I'm finally ready to move on with my life and to pull up the anchor that has distracted my ship. Ella is getting frustrated with me about my reaction to the note. She has been on me to deal with it so we can put it behind us. I know she is right. She's usually way ahead of the curve when it comes to what I need as well as what we as a family need. I tend to listen to Ella; she's a very smart woman.

My first wife Shelly and I were married for twenty-one years. Our marriage was one that formed out of innocence and quite frankly, insecurity. Of course, at the time it seemed perfect. I was on top of the world, and from my limited perspective, she was perfect. In the end, time revealed that she was not. I myself was light years away from maturity and thought that the world was mine for the taking. I was raised on Burt Reynolds and Steve McQueen movies; I felt like I was another giant just waiting to be discovered. It took years of hard work, parenthood and even a few bouts with the law to help me to reach the needed humility to grow up and out of selfishness. I still believe that my dreams and aspirations were relevant, but perspective is the offspring of a well-lived life. When I was young I had a tendency to wear blinders and ignored the debris my actions would leave behind. Shelly was a good woman but we were so different I think it was doomed from the start. She married a young radical while looking for stability. Stability comes down the road with age and insecurity is the anti-venom for success. The first few years were fun but after the honeymoon phase had run its course we ended up faking it for years; to her credit, she stayed with me through my wilder years but eventually, we grew apart. It was Shelly's idea to divorce; I fought her tooth and nail to try to keep our marriage afloat. I guess in the end I would have to say she did us both a favor.

Ella and I both agree that the second marriage gets the benefit of all the mistakes we made in our first. I've learned to appreciate and cherish Ella. I don't really believe I gave Shelly that kind of respect, not on a truly mature level.

Ella has encouraged me to take a couple of days and spent some time alone down at the beach to clear my head. I wanted her to come with me, but she said that she wanted me to go and face my giants head on. She told me to find a quiet spot, sit down and read the note that my dad sent to me before taking his life. She was adamant about it. It was just the push I needed. I agreed and set my sights on the upcoming weekend to hit the beach. I took about a half day that Friday morning before I left to wrap up all the loose ends around the house, yard work etc. I wanted my plate completely clear before heading to the beach. I finished up and stopped in to give my two little ones a kiss and a hug. They were not on the same page about my trip to the beach not including them. I promised a trip for us all very soon and left them with one hundred kisses. They finally came to a good place with it all and wished me a good time.

My son said to me, "If you go by yourself will you get me a new rock for my collection while you're there?"

I told him I would find a really cool one while I was away. I haven't surfed since I was a teenager but as I was leaving my daughter's bedroom she said, "Catch a few waves for me, Daddy."

"Ok, I'll ride a few twenty foot high waves just for you." When I said this she broke out in laughter and said, "You're a funny daddy. Be careful and come back soon."

"I will sweetie, I love you." She gave me another hug and I walked out to the front yard.

Ella was waiting for me next to my motorcycle. I have a black and chrome big Suzuki Boulevard cruiser that most people mistake it for a Harley from a distance. Unfortunately, it doesn't get a lot of miles on it these days. I don't ride with my family on it because I feel it's too dangerous. My outings are reserved for rare occasions like this one. I raced motocross for eight years as a kid so I would say that I am quite capable when it comes to riding. I was able to spend an hour early this morning cleaning it up and making it shine. It really does look awesome.

"I want you to be careful on this thing,'" Ella says as she reaches over to give me one more hug. We have already had a long talk while we had our morning coffee so we are both on board with my going down to the beach alone. I will be staying at the bed and breakfast that Ella and I stay at once a year. It's called The Water's View and is our favorite place to be in the whole world. It overlooks a little sailboat harbor about one and a half miles from New Smyrna Beach.

My ride is starting off nicely; the pipes are loud and roaring at a level that I feel keeps me safe. Cars and trucks on the road are fully aware that I am near due to the custom Vance and Hines pipes that I had put on my bike last year. I crank the throttle up and hit the freeway doing sixty-five miles an hour. It is relatively close to home and only takes just under an hour to get from my house to the beach. The sun will be up for about three more hours so I should be able to get checked into my room and out to the beach well before sundown. The freeway traffic is not bad this afternoon; the wind in my face feels great. Just about ten minutes more and I will be there.

As I cruised down the final stretch of road the reasons for my trip are coming back into view. I know the next couple of days will need to be productive. I'm getting some down time, which is the equivalent of gold these days so I need to make it count. The road feels comfortable, my engine has a smooth hum and the wind blows across my face offering its cool refreshing contribution to this welcome road trip. This memory lane road trip is reigniting past memories and I find myself reminiscing about the old days of my first marriage, my youth. The twisting roads that brought me here are also reminding me of the day I heard the news, the six words that changed my life, the beginning of the end of my innocent life.

Years before Shelly and I divorced, I took a lot of freelance carpentry jobs and was laid on and off for around six years. The pay was good and the work was challenging. Then I landed a really good gig with a television production company. It is a popular kids TV channel, owned by the giant corporation. I've become quite the accomplished carpenter these days. I grew up doing it but the jobs I've had in since leaving Texas, including this place, have stretched my abilities to new heights. Thinking back to the day that transitioned my life is strangely clear, even after all these years.

I was working for Harold in the studio's shop, an odd yet friendly man that I have been blessed to know and work for. He had me making props for the studio on that day, random things for another game show. I don't yet have the measurements for one of the props that I would be making; Harold told me to keep myself busy out in the shop until he was ready for me. To go forward with the build I will have to wait for him to nail down the specs from the studio.

I take some time getting my tools together for the project. While I was waiting I did a quick clean up in the shop; Harold calls me over the intercom to come to his office after about a half an hour with the project information that had been sent over. He wants me to build a rolling table for the prop department at the studios. I have been asked to trim it in six-inch foam and make the foam look like nicely formed molding. This will be fun. I make the table out of speed rail and speed rail fittings. After several hours of fabrication, I had the project ready for paint. It was nice and clean looking. I was proud of it and started rolling it to the paint department so they could work their magic on it.

Harold walked up next to me when I was rolling it to paint. He said, "What took you so long?" I know he was kidding but he always had this serious look on his face that made you feel just a bit south of normal when he was trying to act like the boss. His after-hours look was downright comforting but at work, he took on a strange serious personality. I told him I was seeking perfection and I wanted to make the table perfect. He looked at me with that look that would make the average guy cringe. I knew that he was kidding. He turned and walked off in a different direction without another word. Just as I wheeled the table up to paint Mindy comes out of her office and says to me in a stressed voice that my wife is on the phone and it sounds urgent. I ran across the shop to the phone over by receiving and pick up. Her voice sounds scared. She says something has happened and that I need to come home. I ask her what's going on and she says that I just need to come home. I tell her not to worry that I will be right there.

I ran into Harold's office and tell him that I have an emergency and that I have to leave for the day. He tells me to go and not to worry about it. I ran and grabbed my helmet and ran out to the parking lot. I threw my leg over my red 750 Honda Night Hawk motorcycle and fired it up. I bought it new about a year earlier after a year of riding a smaller 250 Nighthawk for years prior to that. The 750 was fast and reliable. It had great handling. I backed it out of the parking spot and blew out of the parking lot with a twisted throttle and a raging engine.

I'm flying down the road with panic in my heart. There was an emergency at home. Shelly said I needed to come home. Was it my children, was it my parents, or was it a death in the family. What the hell was it? I turn the corner and onto a large overpass that I knew would be the fastest way home. The road was clear and I wasted no time getting the bike into a fast pace. I'm picking up speed and hoping there are no cops in the area. I look down at the speedometer and it reads eighty-five. I twist the throttle a bit further and that's where I heard the pop. It was a strange pulling sound coming from my rear wheel. I didn't have time to look down because it was becoming apparent that my bike was no longer functioning in a normal fashion. The back wheel was locked up and I was beginning to fishtail from side to side. Everything was going so fast and then as if by magic, things went almost silent. I was sliding almost totally sideways without a sound. I could tell things were out of control, yet there was a strange sense of calm that flowed out of my abilities. I have raced motocross, I've plowed down more than my fair share of close calls but something was different. I was sliding almost completely sideways for a long, long time. I should have flipped by now. I was going so fast, yet everything seemed to move in slow motion. It was as if an angel or some supernatural being was holding me in the palm of its hand. I was safe; at least that's how it felt. I was prepared for the worst but the worst was not ready to greet me just yet.

I slid for what seemed like forever. My speed was decreasing and it was becoming clear that I was going to pull this near crash off. My bike came to a halt and I sat there for a few minutes trying to assess what I had just been through. I wondered if the angel that had saved me was still around or not. I had just had a supernatural experience and that was undeniable. I looked up and thanked God. My duffel bag had come off and locked itself in my chain sprocket. My wheel was locked. To free my wheel, I rolled it forward until I could pull out the torn bag. I held up the black bag. It was badly tattered but I decided to keep it for posterity. I put it back in my bungee mesh and started up my red ride. I looked around and noticed that this normally busy John Young road was completely empty. I wondered if that was part of the miracle? If there had been cars I don't know if I could have managed the incident. I still to this day don't fully know if it was my abilities or God that got me through that one. I pulled back onto the road. My back wheel had a flat spot from the long slide. It was so worn that my bike hopped on each wheel revolution. I hopped down the road back home remembering the emergency that seemed to be waiting for me. My mind was racing yet I had an odd calm about me after my sliding experience.

I pulled into my neighborhood to notice several cars in front of my house. There were eight to ten people from my church including my wife and kids standing outside waiting for me. When I pulled into the driveway and the family minister from our church, Max came up to me. I turned the key to my bike off and he asked me to give him my keys. I was so stressed from the ride home that I gladly gave them to him. He held out his hand and I dropped them into his hand. As soon as I saw him put them in his pocket I knew something tragic was unfolding. Everyone's eyes were on me as I swung my leg over and off my motorcycle. The new preacher from our church was there. He was a pretty big man. He said to everyone that we should go inside. My mind was racing as I followed them in. I walked slowly behind everyone not wanting to hear what I was getting ready to hear. I could hear my steps, the birds; I looked back to my bike and torn duffle bag. I walked just into the house and Max walked past me and shut the front door. The foyer was relatively long and narrow and I stopped halfway into it and said, "Tell me." John, the preacher walked up to me and said in his deep powerful voice, "Your father has taken his life."

Those six words would haunt me for years to come. I backed up to the wall and began to press my back into it. I pushed as hard as I can. I wanted to go into the wall and disappear. I must have looked so pitiful, all those eyes on me trying to push myself back into the wall. I don't know how long that lasted but the phone rang. Shelly said it was my step-mom calling from Texas. I ran to the phone and she was sounding completely panicked. She said the police were there and my dad was still in the driveway where he had shot himself. I screamed at her to take the phone over to him, that I wanted him to hear my voice. She wouldn't do it. She said that he followed her out his patio door with a 357 in one hand and his 32 in his back pocket. I think they had just argued, she didn't say that but I knew how things went over there so I could hear it in her voice. In the past, I had heard her even dare my dad to kill himself when they would argue. She said she got in her car to leave and he walked out

112

onto the driveway and raised his hand very nicely and waved goodbye with his fingers. He then put the gun into his mouth and pulled the trigger.

I went down to Texas and buried my dad.

I rode for the next few minutes down the highway heading towards New Smyrna. The old memories are still painful to relive yet they no longer have the paralyzing effect that they used to. I have played that scene out in my head over a thousand times now and after many years have put what I thought was my role in all of it in a safe place. The air feels good on my face. There really is nothing like riding down the open road on a motorcycle. It offers me the psychological freedom that is so elusive in daily life. The day's light is fading though but I still have a couple of hours left before sunset. I want to get checked in and then get over to the beach to watch the sun go down.

The open road is working for me today because I'm riding into New Smyrna with a heart that already feels less heavy, the beach air will do that for a person; the twist of a motorcycle throttle will do that for a person. I smell the salt air and feel it blowing across my face like the grace of God. I turn right and ease down the small road that leads to The Water's View. I look to the left and enjoy the ship channel that runs across the street. It's so beautiful. I take another right turn into the parking lot for The Water's View and find a good spot to park my bike. They have a couple of garages for motorcycles so I will be able to park my bike in one of them tonight.

I'm traveling light on this trip; I've just brought a duffle bag and a pair of flip-flops. I walk up the ramped walkway that leads around the building and onto the front porch. The building is very old yet it has had the benefit of good ownership. When you enter the old plantation style bed and breakfast, it is like stepping back in time. The stairs that go up three stories are made with dark custom woodworking. The lobby has a piano off to the side and the walls are lined with bookshelves. Old yet nicely kept comfortable couches and chairs are placed tastefully about. There are a couple of dining rooms and a serve yourself, a small country kitchen where they keep snacks and a refrigerator filled with cokes and beer. Another room just behind the serving kitchen can be accessed. It is the larger kitchen area where all of the meals are prepared. From the times Ella and I have been here I have come to know that the large kitchen is off limits to the guests. The manager is also the head chef and has no patience for kitchen trespassers. She bit my head off the first time I stayed here for walking in uninvited. After letting me know that the room would always be off limits she then walked me into the serving kitchen, opened the refrigerator and handed me a beer. She smiled and gave me a wink and said that this was my kitchen and that was hers. I told her that sounded fair to me.

I got the keys from the manager who was surprised to see me by myself. I usually call and reserve a room but today I took a chance and just rode over. I really hadn't thought about making a reservation. Ella usually takes care of our reservations when we come over to stay overnight. My mind has been too busy lately. I was in luck because the top floor had a room that faced the harbor. It was perfect. I put a few things away and went back out to put my bike up in the garage. I'm planning on having a few beers tonight so I called a cab to bring me over to the beach. The main street on Flagler Avenue, which is not far from here, is lined with surf shops, gift shops, and pubs. This is where Ella and I like to go when we come down to get away. At the end of the street, there is a restaurant and pub that faces the beach. I think I will get a burger and a few beers. I'll be able to sit out on the deck and watch the sun go down from there. My plan is to spend some time walking down the beach after the sun goes down and then find a quiet spot to read the note that my dad wrote to me.

There is a good breeze coming off the ocean this evening. My waitress is doing a stellar job of getting me food and drinks. The burger I had was humungous, I had sautéed mushrooms on the side and sweet potato fries with brown sugar sprinkled on top. This place is rich with customers this evening. A lot of obvious locals mixed in with the snowbirds and stray travelers. I love an environment with a mixed crowd. It reminds me of the three years I spent in Manhattan. These people are all living out their individual stories, making mistakes and sharing good times. I would prefer that Ella and the kids were here but I know that my time here needs to be purposeful. I wonder what the residents at Blue Lakes are doing tonight? I usually leave the community at about four in the afternoon so I seldom get to see the nightlife that plays out. I look around at the people in the pub and wonder if they know how lucky they are. I can hear the waves as they crash into the beach and I find myself thinking about my dad. I wonder at what point he stopped realizing how lucky he was. Whatever it was that drove him off the cliff would have been a faded memory by now if he would have just held on. The here and now is so much better than old baggage. Memories are good things to have in your psychological toolbox, but what is in front of us is actually reality and still offers choices and surprises. What a shame it is to waste a lifetime being sad due to a brief few moments of time.

My mind was just getting warmed up when my waitress stops by and asks, "Are you ready for some desert?"

I say to her with a smile, "I was hoping that I could order a beer."

She laughs and says, "We've got most any beer your palette desires, what kind would you like?"

"I'm thinking a pint of Bass would be just the thing." She said she would get it for me and then I excused myself to the men's room saying, "I'll be right back, is there a jukebox?"

She replied, "Oh sure, it's right over in the corner next to the ladies restroom. I could use some music, thanks."

After leaving the men's room I stopped by and put in five dollars' worth of music in the jukebox. I picked out a few songs from U2 and some classic Talking Heads and then told my waitress to help herself to all the remaining credits. She was giddy about that. I guess when you're young and at work, music is the ultimate motivator. She is good at her job though because when I returned to my table, a cold pint of Bass was waiting for me.

I sipped my beer and listened to the music while staring out to sea. The sun went down offering its photon gifts in an unending supply of tints and hues. I looked across the ocean and wondered if someone on the other side could be sitting in a café or pub doing the exact same thing. I wondered if that beer that they were enjoying tasted as good as mine. I wondered if the buzz flooded their mind with memories and dreams the way mine is. I spend the next hour sipping several beers and watching the nightlife on the beach and in the pub. I touch my front pocket to make sure that I still have the note and find that it is there safe and sound. It's been searching for me for the past fifteen years. It waited at the bottom of an old photo album for years and years to be read. Its patient words were now anxious to get out into reality. Tonight I will put an end to the years of questions and anxieties. I down the rest of my beer and pay my tab. I have enjoyed my waitress's table for the past couple of hours so I make sure to leave her a healthy tip. I stand up and head out towards the beach. I feel pretty good, the meal was great and I've got a small beer buzz, which has taken the edge off. I feel relaxed; I feel more relaxed than I have felt in years. This was a great idea to come down here and have some time to myself to relax and find some clarity.

The sand is packed hard on the shoreline as it meets the incoming waves; the sound of the ocean is like a roaring lion. I think heaven sounds like the beach at night. That's about as good of a guess as anything else I can imagine. I look up and see nothing but stars in this Florida night. The wind is just cold enough to keep me from wandering straight out into the ocean. I'm thinking tomorrow morning I will be out there, but tonight just the sights and sounds will be sufficient. I remember my dad and how he was when I was a kid; he loved the ocean; his face was always sunburned and made fishing a priority in our lives. He was a hardworking man and he taught me to be the same way. He was also a drinking man; not like the few beers I had tonight but multiple beers and whiskey on most occasions. He would work from daylight to sunset most of the week but in the last few years of his life, he had made a good bit of money, which freed him up to fish and hunt and bar hop a lot more. He had a boat and a bay house next to the Gulf of Mexico. We spent most of my early teenage years fishing and riding motorcycles in that bay house's small fishing town neighborhood. It was in Annuack, Texas, a great place to breathe fresh air and slow down a few paces.

My dad drank most of his beer in The Whiskey Stop. It was a small, hole in the wall beer joint about a mile down the road from where we lived. He knew everyone there. The place could get quite rowdy late at night and fights were a regular occurrence; I often feared for my dad's safety when he would sit at the bar and order round after round. He was raised with eleven brothers and one sister.

My grandpa was quite the rebel; I never met him because he died before I was born. He had one hundred acres of farmland and a still deep in his woods so my dad had plenty of exposure to a rough and ready country life. Dad knew how to handle himself in a place like this. I would go down and play pool with him when I was a teenager. They would serve me a beer even though I wasn't of age. In a place like that, the cops looked the other way; that was the way it was in a lot of places where I grew up back in Texas. Nowadays with a camera at every red light and zero tolerance for most things, life is completely different. Some of it has changed for the better, but freedom is, in my opinion, has come to look like a frog in a pot of cold water, sitting on the stove. The frog will stay in the water as it heats up and will not even try to escape, that an odd thing to know. The burner is on and the cameras are watching. Wow, that's a whole different thing, my mind is all over the map. I guess that's why I have put off dealing with this note from my dad. It brings up a lot of old memories that I have worked so hard to put behind me.

It was dark but I had my trusty flashlight on my belt so I knew I would be able to read out here on the beach. I've walked about a mile down the beach now and I am alone. I sit in the sand and take out the note, staring at the envelope that has been waiting all these years to be read. I look up and whisper in the air, "I'm here Dad, what is it that you wanted to say? I'm sorry it took me so long to get to a place that I could read your note. Before I begin reading I want you to know that I'm so mad at you for what you did. You've put a stain on my heart that will never go away. I know you had your reasons, but you've really hurt me, Dad."

I turn the head of my flashlight and the illuminated envelope is in view. The letter had tape on the back of it. The adhesive was no longer guarding its treasure, only the tape that was stuck so well it forced me to rip the top section of the paper to get to the letter; I slowly pull out what were my dad's final thoughts and intentions. The note inside appeared to have been crinkled up and then smoothed out, When I unfolded the note to be read my thoughts raced; my heart was moving with fast paced beats; the black penned words came into full view. My dad then went on to reveal himself to me fifteen years after he took his life.

Earl, I want you to know that I love you and have enjoyed having you as my son. You are a special man and I have always loved watching you take a path less traveled. I loved watching you ride your dirt bike when you were little. I loved having you by my side at work. We had a good run but now I'm going to have to go somewhere. I will be ending my time here on this earth and I hope you can forgive me. I hope God can forgive me. I tried to call you but you were not home. I wanted to say goodbye I don't know any other way to fix my problem. I don't think it can be fixed or I would have already done what needed to be done. I will be taking my life. I have a problem. Your stepmother doesn't get it and I cannot face it anymore without action. It is something I have to do and I want you to know that it is not your fault. It is not something that I can or want to burden you with. I couldn't stand to have this affect you and your family so I have to go. I want nothing more than for you and your family to have a good life. Enjoy our memories together and tell everyone that cares to ask that I am sorry for everything. Earl, I have a problem. I have left a phone number and a name for you to call. It is on the backside of this letter. I left something with them for you. Please call them soon because it will not be there for long I fear. I love you; be a good boy, goodbye.

I stared at the letters and words, thoughts in a daze. Tears and anger poured out of my eyes like a broken faucet. I started to shake and could not decipher my emotions. I was trembling with a bubbling rage. After about two minutes of trying to suppress the pressure, I stood up and screamed at the top of my lungs, "DAD!" I yelled at the black sky, "What fucking problem! DAD, where the hell did you go?" I continued to yell and rage for what seemed like another half hour, in reality, it was only minutes. I fell to the ground and went silent, laying face up in the sand.

After so many years I get a note that tells me not much more than I already knew. I knew my dad loved me. We were two peas in a pod for the better part of my life. What the hell was his problem and why would it cause him to take his life? I tried to relax; I took several large breaths and exhaled out as slowly as I could. I sat up then continued sitting for at least an hour calming my thoughts. The name and phone number that my dad had written on the back of the note had been scribbled out and I could not make out any of it. That is completely screwed. Someone has hidden the phone number and name from me. I guess it could have been my stepbrother or a number of people who had access to the note. It's been fifteen years now and the information that my dad had left for me is gone anyway I'm sure. Wow, that's messed up. I don't care. I'm choosing to let it go.

After a few more minutes I start getting a peace that I haven't had for weeks, even years. I got to read his words. He told me all he could, and I had to let that be enough. After so many years I had the privilege of a few more words from my dad and that to me was worth a pot of gold. He was a good man. I know he was a rebel but that's one of the characteristics that made him so special to me. Whatever problem he had, it is over now. I wish he would have had the courage to get help and fight through whatever his problem was but it's too late for wishing. It's over.

I've had a long forty-nine years of life; I've learned so much and made more than my fair share of mistakes. In my youth, my dad was there for me and offered me grace. In my manhood, I will do the same for him. I love him and I always will. I stand up and look into the night sky and gaze at its calming powerful stars. Someday I will not be here either and that's just fine with me. While I'm here I will not be frightened or timid; this short life is tricky but no match for the human spirit. Ella and the kids count on me and with the time I have left here on earth I will live largely and lead my family. I kneel down in the sand and say a prayer for my dad and thank my God for his grace. The wind blows on my face as I raise my face up to the sea; I open up my eyes and stare at its vastness. The waves come in with a crashing roar just as they do when it is light; giving gifts to everything it touches. The moon hangs low and lights up the oceans dark waters and creating a beautiful site to see. The two dance together as if they were old friends. This night is good.

I walk back up the beach towards the pub that helped to begin this journey. After about twenty minutes of walking, I reach the front door and peek inside through the pub's window. I see my waitress still scurrying about serving drinks. I walk in and see that my chair from before is just getting ready to become available once again. A man and woman are just getting up. The man looks over at the waitress and holds up the cash for his check.

She waves at him and says thanks. I sit back at my table and am once again greeted by the waitress as she says, "Back for round two?"

"I am ready for round two. Let's make it a Black n Tan this time," I say with a grin.

"Yummy, I'll be right back with your drink."

I look around and the place is jumping. The music is playing loud and everyone seems to be enjoying themselves. It's funny how life goes on and on. Trouble comes and trouble goes, but one thing I've come to recognize is the fact that trouble and sorrow are temporary. I realize tonight that the worries of the world are only as powerful as we let them become. The letter has been read now and whatever was at the end of his final message concerning the phone number is gone. I will no longer give it the power to rule my thoughts. I have Ella and the kids and a great job at Blue Lakes. Those residents are still alive and kicking and they are my extended family. Life is short and for the first time in months, I feel light again.

The waitress brings me my Black and Tan and says, "There are about three credits on the jukebox if you're interested. What comes around goes around."

I smile and say, "That sounds good to me; it's a great jukebox with plenty of songs an old guy like me can still recognize."

She winks at me in with a sexy smile and leans into my ear and says, "Experience is sexy." She smiles and leaves me with a grin. I'm feeling so relieved to have the burden of my dad's note finally behind me; I feel like myself again. I sit and enjoy a couple more beers and some music. I call a cab and make my way back to the bed and breakfast. I'm ready to get snuggled up in the room. Tomorrow I'll ride my motorcycle down to the beach and enjoy the day before heading back home.

I get back to The Water's View safe and sound. The front of the building has a large wrap around porch with rocking chairs and a porch swing that is very comfortable. I sit down in one of the wicker rocking chairs and look out into the starlit darkness of the waterway. There is no one else out front but for me. I guess it is pretty late; I think it's after midnight. I watch the sailboats that are tied off just off the shore in the water. They rock from side to side ever so slowly as the breeze periodically moves the waves. I sit and enjoy the most peaceful sights and sounds I've enjoyed in years and slowly fall asleep right where I sit.

The sun is just coming up as my eyes open. I realize that I snuggled up in the rocking chair for a good night's sleep. I can smell the coffee brewing from the front lobby just inside from where I spent my night. I get up and stretch my back out some to get the creaks out. Even though the chair was comfortable, it was still a chair. I feel pretty rested anyway. I'm not used to having as many beers as I did so that most likely helped me to be relaxed enough to not mind sleeping in a chair. I walk in to get a cup of coffee. That's one of the things that I love about this place is the fresh coffee that is ready for the guests the better part of every day. I pour myself a cup and walk back outside to enjoy the first cup of the day while watching the sun come up.

After a shower, some breakfast and a little more rest I pay my bill and head out. Once my bike is packed up again I swing my leg over the seat and get comfortable. I strap my helmet on and hit the start button to engage my bike's eager engine. I let it warm up for a couple of minutes and then slowly pull out on the street heading towards the beach. It's only ten thirty in the morning so the sun is just now working its magic on the day. It's getting warmer and the people are starting to move about the quiet streets in their baggy shorts and bathing suits. I'm enjoying the sound of my bike as it moves along with a confident hum. I'm back in the saddle again and it's a beautiful day. I head towards Flagler Avenue to go to the gift shops before I do anything else. I want to get my son a new rock for his collection and something for my little girl as well. I cruise down the back roads that lead towards the beach and quickly arrive. New Smyrna is looking good today; Flagler Avenue is full of locals, tourists, and plenty of places to shop. I ease down the road enjoying the sights and smells of all the restaurants I pass. I rev my engine to accommodate two small boys with their parents giving me two thumbs up. One of them yells out to me, "I like your bike!"

Life is good.

Baby Winters

My trip to the beach was just what I needed to get back in the groove and to start forward thinking again. I was feeling like my old self and relating to the residents at Blue Lakes as I did in the earlier days when I started. Thankfully I'm past the germ-a-phobic stage and can now give myself more fully to my job. I want to be more instrumental in helping the residents through their transitional stages, or at least try to understand them better so I can communicate more on their level. Yes, I know that my job is keeping the building's maintenance in order and running the housekeeping department, but I feel a higher calling. I want to matter in this day-to-day life. We never know how much time we have so given all we have seems appropriate. Working with the people in memory care centers is not like any other place. You can't ignore what's happening around you and believe me, there is plenty going on around you.

Baby Winters, one of our residents, has gone into a new phase or level in her Alzheimer's. The plastic doll that she held was the love of her life and in her mind, nothing short of truly alive. The other associates and I knew to treat Miss Baby's doll with kid gloves. It was an important key to keeping her content; for several weeks before the doll was introduced we noticed that Miss Baby had gone downhill in her motor skills and her speech patterns were getting irregular. She took to moaning and whimpering on an ongoing basis. She would cry out that she needed to go home or she needed her yellow bike. She would walk the entire building from one end to another constantly yelling out that she wanted to go home. She would stand by the front door and stare out as if waiting for her ride. "Where's my yellow bike!" That was the phrase I remember the most; it was getting so bad that we could no longer allow her to be with the rest of the residents because she would upset the others with her constant whimpering and extreme yelling. She was not trying to be disruptive; in her mind, she knew what she wanted, but when the staff would try to console her she would quickly get louder and louder.

Thankfully all of that changed. I remember the day the activities director came in with a newly purchased baby doll. It was a girl doll in pink clothing and big blue eyes. It was love at first sight for Miss Baby and her new baby doll. She was almost immediately transformed into a nurturing state. She must have longed for a time when she herself was a mother, or maybe she never even had children, I honestly never knew. It was the medicine she needed though. How ironic that this lady's name was really Baby. I suppose it could've been a nickname from way back, but that's the name she came in with, Baby Winters. She had progressed to the many stages of Alzheimer's right before our eyes. The progression was at times hard to watch. She would stay at a certain level and you would begin to think that that was how it would be and then without notice, she would transition to another stage. The transitions seemed to be escalating more quickly these days. The plastic baby had come to represent her own child. She talked to it, protected it, and loved it with everything she had. She had retained her natural sense of humor and wit through the course of her time with us here at Blue Lakes; just when you thought her mind was going downhill she would interject herself into the middle of someone's conversation and say something completely poignant and relevant to what they were saying. That always fascinated me. It taught me to never write any one of our residents off, not that I or anyone else would, but I could never tell where they were at in their dementia because the stages would sometimes overlap leaving one skill behind while another set of skills were sharp as a steak knife. I suspect the nurses higher up the food chain had a better handle on what level she was at, but I'm a handyman, not a nurse. I do pay attention though.

When I would arrive in the mornings soon after she had received her new baby, she would be sitting in one of the lobby chairs next to the front door. When I would enter the building she greeted me with the same thing most every morning; she would say, "It's about time you got back here."

"Yes ma'am," I would say to her, "How's the kid?"

"Oh she's just fine, she cried most of the night but she seems fine now."

Her versions of how the night went would vary from day to day but our conversations always started out the same. It was like being in my own version of the movie Groundhog Day with Bill Murray. It was a pleasant way to come into work each day. Time went on and Baby Winters continued in her transitions; we were all happy to have her with us. She brought us hope in seeing that we were able to help her through her crying stage and into the role of a mother. Who knows, maybe the cure is right around the corner. Maybe it will be revealed and brought out of the darkness and into the Light. I think it will.

Win a Handyman

The drawing was to be done this afternoon by one of the family members of our community. I asked Ronnie, the son of one of our residents to do the drawing primarily because he was so vocal about not needing a handyman because he already was one. He was actually a funny guy. He told a lot of stories to the staff about his mom when he came to visit her. He seemed nervous and I'm thinking a bit embarrassed about his mom's condition. People all have their individual reaction to their family's memory loss. It's understandable. Nobody wants to go through it but choices are sent out across the cosmos on a daily basis. They land on us wherever we are and we deal with them how only we can.

I wanted to do something that would have an impact on our efforts to raise research money for the development of cures for the Alzheimer's disease. Our management team was trying to come up with ideas to raise money for the cause. It occurred to me that I could raffle myself off as a handyman. Why not? Everyone has things broken around the house or unfinished projects that no one has time to get back to. Everyone at work seemed to think it was a great idea so I went with it. I had delusions of grandeur when it came to how it would be received. For such a great idea I was sure I would have to purchase endless amounts of raffle tickets. I thought I would raise thousands of dollars for the cause; indeed I went as far as to brag that my effort would bring in a minimum of a thousand dollars in ticket sales.

Not so much. After making my spill to the staff and selling about fifteen tickets I soon realized that my great idea was just that, a great idea. To make it take off I would have to get off my butt and market it to people within the community as well as out in the surrounding neighborhoods. I would need to attend functions and set up tables at the local fairs and things along those lines. This is what I should have done, not what I did. I'm ashamed to admit it but quite frankly I let it go. When I didn't get bombarded with ticket sales right away I sort of lost interest. The months rolled by and I would sell the occasional ticket but that was pretty much it. I had set a date very early on for the winning raffle ticket to be drawn and today was the day. This afternoon I would have Ronnie pull the winning ticket out and I could then perform my free handyman day for the winner and move on with my moneymaking tale between my legs. To date I have raised a hundred and seventy dollars in ticket sales; I should be at least slightly proud of that but the fact that I put so little effort into it was embarrassing. Ronnie and several of the staff were present for the drawing. Mrs. Whitfield, the staff, and even Ronnie gave me a lot of praise for my efforts. He said he was proud of me for putting myself out there to raise money. I guess it is a good thing but when you know you can do better it's always hard, at least for me, to accept the praise when I know I could've done more.

He reaches in our large glass bowl that we had housing the tickets and pulled out a winner. With about ten of us at the drawing, the applause was loud and the cheers were well provided.

Ronnie read out the name loud and clear for everyone to hear, "Today's winner for Mr. Hadley's 'Win a Handyman' is Anna Kelly!"

He immediately began clapping with only a couple of other associates joining in. Most of the rest of us just stood there with our jaws tight and our heads slowly dropping downward. Mr. Kelly, one of our community's residents, had just passed away not two days before the drawing. He had been with us for six years and was the favorite resident at Blue Lakes, hands down of most any associate you could ask. He was our mascot if that's not too inappropriate to say.

When you thought of our community and any function you thought about Mr. Kelly. He had come to us very early in his dementia and stayed with us through the many stages of his Alzheimer's disease. He knew of his memory problems early on and had the means and where with all to set himself up to move into our community when it became clear that he could no longer take care of himself. From what I had heard he wasn't married. He had a daughter that came only twice a year to visit him according to the head nurse. I always thought it was odd that she came so infrequently since I had heard that she lived literally right down the street. She was at the Halloween party with her dad but she didn't stay very long from what I remembered. She came in a few weeks ago to see him; that's when she bought the handyman raffle ticket from me. I think she was just being polite when she bought it; she handed me a five-dollar bill from her purse, which was worth three tickets. After filling out her name and phone number on the by she smiled, said thank you and left soon afterward. I guess that's how it goes with raffles; you never know who will win. Since Mr. Kelly passed away only two days ago I thought I would give it a couple of weeks before calling to allow the family time to grieve.

I've seen families go through the passing of their loved ones since starting here and it tends to go pretty well. By the time they've had their family members stay here and watched them go through memory loss and Alzheimer's they can see it is better that they do pass on and into a better place. After Alzheimer's does its full damage to a person's life, it is better served in the spirit realm as far as I'm concerned. It's an awful thing to watch, but the great thing about where I work is it allows these people to pass on with dignity.

I removed all the raffle signs and took the three posters down that I had put up. There was a kind of hole left in our community over the next couple of weeks. It's like I said, Mr. Kelly was a big part of everything we did here. He had a funny laugh that he would belt out periodically during our group functions. He was a very happy man, which is not always the case with most of our residents. He seemed to adapt from one stage to the next in his disease with a gentle spirit. He laughed a lot. Something I think I learned from him is that laughing is the best medicine there is. Mr. Kelly had a contagious spirit that will be missed in our community. He was a gift.

I waited three weeks to call his daughter. I tried to get the nerve to call after two weeks but I thought another week would be better. It's not a conversation that can be planned in my opinion; I decided to just call, offer my condolences and see how it goes. The phone rang for four rings, and I decided to let it ring until her voicemail picked up so I could leave her a message.

After the fifth ring, a woman answered, and I said, "Hello Mrs. Kelly, this is Earl Hadley; we met a few weeks ago at Blue Lakes where your dad was staying."

There was a short pause on her end, "Hello."

"I'm so sorry about your dad; how are you doing?"

"I'm doing ok" she replied, "Thank you for asking; how can I help you, Earl?"

"You bought a raffle ticket from me a few weeks back when you were visiting your dad; I wanted to let you know that you won the contest, you were the winner."

"That's funny, I forgot about the drawing. I won?"

"Yes ma'am you did, you won."

"That's very nice, what was it you were doing with this? I remember something about handyman work?"

"Yes ma'am, I will be spending a day taking care of any chores you need to be done around the house; this can also include small carpentry projects or plumbing projects. I have all the tools to take care of most anything. If you decide you want shelving built or installed, I just ask that you provide the building materials. Basically, I will take care of anything around the house free of any labor charges."

She said she would have to think about what she might need and that she would like to call me back with a few ideas. I told her to take her time, that this would be an open-ended prize. I told her that we all missed her dad and I'm sure she was still going through a lot with his passing. She was noticeably short with her conversation; I imagine losing her dad was devastating. I wondered about the fact that she visited him so infrequently knowing she lived so close. Every family has their reasons and their own secrets. Hers were none of my business. I know this handyman prize is a good idea; I just didn't picture it like this. My life, indeed everyone's life is full of twists and turns and all tend to unravel into the unexpected. At my age, almost forty-nine now, I have learned that we get what we need, and sometimes a little of what we want gets mixed in for good measure.

Mrs. Kelly called me about a week and a half later. I was at home about seven in the evening; my family and I were just sitting down for dinner. I took her call anyway which is actually rare for me to do at dinnertime, but something told me I should.

When I answered she asked in a quiet voice, "Hello Earl, I'm sorry for calling so late in the day; can you talk about your contest now or this not a good time?"

She seemed nervous, I was glad she called; I was beginning to think she was going to take a pass on the whole thing. "Mrs. Kelly, we are just sitting down for dinner, can I call you back in an hour?"

She said that would be fine: she told me to take my time and that if I needed to call back tomorrow that would be fine. During dinner, I told my wife who it was and she encouraged me to call her back right after we were finished eating. She said this was probably awkward for her; I could tell by Mrs. Kelly's demeanor on the phone that it was. I did call her back after we ate and she said she had thought about what I had said about shelving. She said her garage could use some shelving if I would like to put them in for her. After getting an idea of what was going up on then I got an idea of her tastes and expectations of how it should look. She said her garage was a three-car garage; she asked if I could use wood instead of wire shelving. She said the wire shelving seemed very clinical; I agreed with her on that. She said that she would be glad to buy whatever materials I might need. She said she would be painting them herself white after I was finished. Woodworking is one of my better skills. I decided to really go the extra mile with her shelving and make them sturdy and beautiful. I most always have the mindset when building something for someone that what I build will outlast me and someone will be using it for many years after I'm gone. It's my way of achieving a touch of immortality or at least an abbreviated version of it.

We met a few days later on a Friday evening and bought everything we needed for the project. I was pleased to see she had relaxed some and seemed more at ease with me. She said I was easy to talk to. That's girl code for I'm not the stereotypical man who spends his time watching football. Actually, I like to watch football but I also find it easy to engage in conversation. I'm a weird man in that regard. She met me out in front of the store and drove a sleek, fairly new, silver Lexus. I was impressed by her taste in cars; my van probably looked a little rough parked next to her car. That's not a problem; it is clean and runs great and has some age to it. Old is good in my book; that's my story and I'm sticking to it. Mrs. Kelly was very pleasant.

She must have sensed my comparison of our two cars because she said jokingly, "Do you want to trade?"

I told her no thanks; old vans really do it for me so I could understand why she would want my ride. She smiled. We spent about an hour picking out materials. I already knew what I needed but I wanted to spend some time with Mrs. Kelly so we could get to know each other a little bit. I wanted her to feel comfortable with me. After buying everything we needed, I took the materials home with me to pre-cut some of the wood.

I figured I would set up a table and do all the assembly and finish work at her place so she could enjoy the fact that she was getting something special. I found myself really enjoying all of this because I liked her dad. Mr. Kelly would have appreciated my doing this for his daughter. He used to look up and the contest posters and laugh. I had a picture of myself on the poster carrying ten different tools in my arms for comedic effect. He and everyone who saw it got a kick out of that. I used to say to Mr. Kelly, "Hey boss, am I doing a good job?" He would burst out in that weird laugh of his.

I told Mrs. Kelly, I would call her in about a week once I had a chance to cut up the parts; after that, we could then set a day for me to come over. We had another resident pass this morning. It was expected though. I was glad to see her move on. She had lost most all of her functions and had basically become bedridden for the past month. When I first started working here it would really get me down when someone passed. As time has gone by, I have come to understand that it is inevitable with Alzheimer's, and it really is a blessing. I know there will be a cure someday, but for now, we are all just giving it our best shot with what we have to work with.

I was finished with Mrs. Kelly's shelving parts. I wanted to save the rest of the work to do at her house so I called Mrs. Kelly and was pleased to find out that this coming Saturday will work great for both of our schedules. I went to sleep late that Friday night thinking about what I should say if anything, about her dad's passing. Maybe I should show up as a basic handyman and keep my mouth shut. I guess what needs to be said, if anything, will work itself out naturally. I haven't ever heard Mrs. Kelly mention her husband. I don't even know if she is married. Actually, I don't know anything about her; what if she's some kind of serial killer lady who stalks and preys on handymen? Ok, time to go to sleep; my mind is a bit silly and strange before going to sleep. I reach over and kiss my wife on her shoulder. She is already sleeping but I stare at her as my mind settles down. I am lucky.

I arrive at the gated entrance to Mrs. Kelly's neighborhood. What a beautiful place. The gate is ornate cast iron and is at least twenty feet in height; the landscaping is top of the line. I can't say I would want to pay the electric bill on the large homes that are inside this exclusive neighborhood, but you can't help but admire the time, effort and artistry that has gone into their construction. The people who live in a place like this most likely have worked many hours to become so successful. Success is victory and to be admired. I never played into the class warfare that you see coming from the politicians and those like them. It makes no sense. If there weren't people with money there would not be jobs. I never had a homeless man give me a good paying job. Working at Blue Lakes has helped me to see people on a more level playing field. We have ex-CEOs of large corporations and schoolteachers who taught for thirty years. Everyone gets to the end of life with what they showed up with. We are all just working on the stuff in-between.

I show my ID to the guard at the gate and he hands me a one-page map of the area that has Mrs. Kelly's house location marked so can find it. It takes me about ten minutes to find her house; it was deep in the neighborhood. All the homes were quite large and all off on their own good-sized piece of property. I pulled into the driveway with a sigh of relief for having remembered to bring a piece of thick cardboard to put under my van in case it dropped a few drops of oil as it is prone to do. An oil spot would not be ok in this driveway.

As I pull in Mrs. Kelly's garage door is opening. She comes out and tells me to park right in front of one of the garage doors. There are three bays, one for her car, one for an older motorcycle that I can't yet figure out what make and model it is, and the last one full of what looks like a few piles of random furniture, some tools, and family stuff. There were also a few boxes that looked like they had been around for a good while. The motorcycle was very intriguing. It sat in the middle of its own bay with a powerful presence despite its obvious old age. When I got out of my van and said hello I went right over to the bike. I had to get a better look; I am a motorcycle fan from way back. I raced motocross for eight years as a kid; counting the 2005 Suzuki Boulevard in my garage, I've had over seven kinds of motorcycles since I was a small boy. This bike was amazingly clean. It was Metal Flaked Sunrise Orange, a Honda CB 350. It was the first one of its kind introduced to America in 1968. I don't know that much about historic bikes but I do know Hondas since that's what I grew up riding.

I told Mrs. Kelly that I was so impressed. She thanked me and told me it was her dad's bike. He bought it from one of his buddies that he served with in the Korean War. He would wash or at least rub a cloth on this bike pretty much every day just before he moved into Blue Lakes. He knew his memory was failing but this bike seemed to remind him of everything he wanted to remember. I could relate to that. That's what motorcycles do for me as well.

"Did you ever ride this with him?" I asked.

"Are you kidding me?" she said, "I've ridden this bike with my dad hundreds of times. He and I rode it most every weekend when I was growing up. It wasn't a question of if we were going to ride; it was where we going. My dad and I would search for burger joints and malt shops weeks ahead of time and plan out our trips to get to each one."

I said, "You guys were really close."

"Yes, we were. We still are," she replied.

She smiled nervously and told me to make myself at home. I asked her for some time to get my tools out and to get set up for the project. She said, "I'll check in with you in a little while, use the intercom over on that column if you need to reach me. I can hear it most anywhere in the house."

"Sounds good," I said; it didn't take long for me to get set up and assemble the parts I had already prepared before arriving.

Mrs. Kelly came out about an hour later carrying a tray with cold water and grapes and said, "Here you are Mr. Hadley."

I thanked her and took a second to enjoy her reaction to my work.

"I love it; you are really talented," she said with an honest sincerity.

I told her everything was ready to be mounted to her walls; I just needed to know exactly where we would be putting them. After about an hour I had it all up, secured and looking great. I noticed all the boxes and asked her if that was what she wanted to go on the shelving.

She said, "All the cardboard boxes are not important; I would like to put the things from that box up on your new shelves." She points to an old wooden crate, "It's full of old gadgets and things that were important to my dad. I'm not going to just leave his life in a box stuck up in the attic."

I noticed that she was becoming emotional and said, "No of course not; now you've got new shelves to put some of his stuff on. If you would like, I would be happy to help you."

She said appreciatively, "Are you sure, you've already done so much; I don't want to take advantage of your time. The contest was limited to a day and we've already met at the store to get the materials. You've more than honored your end of the handyman prize."

I replied to her, saying "I'm more than happy to help you with some of the organizing. I liked your dad; I know this will be hard for you. My dad passed away eight years ago and I doubt there is a day that goes by that I don't think of him. It's really hard in the beginning when everything is fresh and nobody knows how to talk about it."

"It is," she said.

I tell her that one of the things that bothered me the most about my dad's passing is that nobody wanted to talk about him anymore. Having his presence just wiped off the face of the earth seemed terrible. He deserved to have his memory stick around. I guess people just don't know what to say. Mrs. Kelly told me that I was the only one so far that has been able to talk with her. "Maybe it's because we don't really know each other. Maybe that's why I feel more comfortable talking about my dad; not that we really have, but I know what you mean about the others involved with my dad's passing."

I told her we should unpack the crate and get some of the things out and up on the wall so they could breathe again. "Let's put some of your favorite things on the shelf and I want you to tell me about a few of them. It'll be fun."

"Fun, Mr. Hadley, you need to get out more." She smiled and appeared to relax.

"Please, call me Earl," I said.

"Ok Earl I will, my name is Anna, and you don't have to call me Mrs. Kelly anymore. Besides, it would be Ms. Kelly if you were going to call me that. I'm not married."

"Oh, ok I wasn't sure, I've been married for almost four years now myself. It's good stuff, I recommend it."

She smiled and said, "I was married once for about three months but that's a whole story in itself. Let's get this crate opened."

"Absolutely," I said, realizing it was a good point in the conversation to move on.

I pulled the screws out quickly from the crate's lid with my screw gun. As Anna opened the lid I watched her face; it was full of emotions that ranged from excited to sad. There was a maroon colored crushed velvet material that covered the contents of the crate. Anna pulled it back to reveal her dad's treasures. She said that before her dad moved into Blue Lakes, she and her dad went to his house and gathered up a few things to pack away. She then paid a man to build a crate to keep it all together and safe until she decided what would become of her and her dad's favorite belongings.

144

"He told me to remember him through these things. He made me promise that after he died I would look them over occasionally and think of him. He also made me promise that I would not be sad when it was his time to go. I don't think I've been able to keep that part of the bargain."

"You will, I said; just give it some time."

I picked up a yellow colored rock. "What's this?"

"Oh be careful, that'll make you invisible!" She had the biggest grin on her face.

"What do you mean?" I asked.

"It's magic!" she said.

"Of course it is; how silly of me," I laughed.

She then went on to say, "When I was about eight years old I was introduced to the magic rock man. That's what I called him. He was a friend of my dad. They served together in the Korean War. We used to ride over to his house at least once a week on my dad's motorcycle. I never knew his name; he was the magic rock man. He would always have a bottle of Coke in his refrigerator for me when we got there. I don't think they sell them anymore; it was back when they used real glass. It was a small bottle, maybe six ounces and the best tasting Coke ever made. This man had thousands of rocks in his house. There would be some in boxes and some out on his workbenches where he would polish them. I guess it was a hobby or maybe a business he was doing, I don't remember. One day we were over at his house and I pointed up to the top of one of his shelves to the rock you're holding. The man told me I had to be careful."

He looked over at my dad and said, "Do you think she is ready to see a rock like that?"

My dad told him it would be ok, but for me to be very careful. I swore that I would. The man gently handed it to me and warned me not to rub it on my skin because it would make me invisible for three hours. He then pulled a cloth out from his desk and told me to keep it wrapped up when carrying it so my hands would not become invisible. Earl, I believed this was real. I believed I had been given ownership of a truly magical rock. For the next few months, I was mesmerized by the power I now had with the rock. I would go into my room and slowly rub the rock all over my body and then sneak out and roam the house and our neighborhood completely invisible. My dad was so bad, Earl. He would see me coming out of my room and call out my name as though I was invisible."

"Anna," he would call out, "I can hear your footsteps but you must have used that pesky rock again because I can't see you." I have run that scene around in my head for the last thirty-five years. He was so great."

I pulled a pair of old binoculars out of the crate; "And this?"

"My dad used them in Korea. He had a lot of military things that he brought back from the war. He had a large chest at the end of his bed that he kept his things in. I wasn't allowed to open the chest.

My dad made it clear to me that some things in life were private and that was one of them. When I was a kid I called this the war chest. It was a summer afternoon when I finally got the courage to peek inside. I was playing in the house. I remember running up and down the hallway and each time I would pass my dad's room the war chest would catch my attention. I had thought about looking at it for years but today curiosity got the best of me. My dad came in early from work one day unexpected. I didn't think I was any danger of being discovered because I had only had the magic rock for a few days at that point and I had just rubbed it all over myself before peeking into the war chest, I had the rock in my hand at that point.

My dad came in and must have been caught off guard by seeing me fascinated with all his special things. He looked right at me for about a minute, not saying a word. I wasn't worried because I knew I was invisible. He must have known what I was thinking because I remember him looking right at the rock in my hand.

He looked in the direction of my bedroom and called out, "Anna, are you home?"

I tiptoed across the hall to my bedroom door and opened my door very surprised to see him home. "Oh hi Dad, when did you get here?"

"Just now," he said, "What are you up to this afternoon?"

"Oh, not much, just playing."

"That's good, I've got some work to do in my office, come see me after dinner, ok?"

"Yes sir," I said."

"So what happened when you went to see him?" I asked.

"He told me that he had something to show me; I followed him to his bedroom. He said he was going to let me see some of his things in the chest; he told me that he would trust me to never look at them again without his special permission. I promised that I would never look in the chest without asking him first. He told me to open the lid so I reached out with overwhelming anticipation. I think my hands were shaking because he told me to relax and it would be ok. I opened the lid and was completely blown away by all of his things. I had not had time earlier in the day to really look since my dad had come home early from work. He had pictures of some of the men he served with, there were a couple of guns and a knife that was big and scary and then there was this."

Anna reached down into the crate near the bottom and pulled out an old tortoiseshell box full of old pictures. "It was the box he kept all his favorite photos in from his time in the service. I will never forget how exciting it was to actually hold it for the first time. It is made of real tortoise shell; it's so beautiful. He took out an old photograph of his dad and showed it to me. I had seen only a couple of photos of my grandfather so this was a real treat. He then took out an old camera from one of his drawers in his room and he took my picture holding the box. "Look, here it is."

Anna pulled back the cloth in the box and showed me the picture she had just described. "He gave it to me a year or so before his dementia started to become obvious. It has been in my living room for years but after my dad moved into Blue Lakes it was too hard to look at so I put it in this crate." She started to cry.

I was feeling awkward but I gave her some time to get it out, saying, "It's good to cry." I busied myself at picking up my tools and started to clean up my work area. I hate when people tell you not to cry. People cry when they need to. It is the best way to release pain in hard times. She collected her composure and apologized for getting so emotional.

"It's ok Anna, it's good to remember your dad and he would have wanted you to remember all of the things he taught you and what he did for you. Memories are one of life's tools."

"That's a good one Earl, did you make that up?"

"Yes just now, it was spontaneous I guess," I laughed nervously.

She smiled and thanked me for coming over. "I'll finish putting the rest of the things on the shelves. My plan is to take a lot of this stuff into one of the rooms in my house. I'm going to create a kind of gallery to display it all. I'm going to put my dad's motorcycle in there as well."

"Sounds like a plan; did you see the picture we had of your dad from the Halloween party? It was priceless."

"I did see that one; that was such a great party. I was only able to stay for an hour because of a prior commitment, but I remember my dad having a really good time. I loved how Blue

Lakes went the extra mile for the holidays; I just couldn't get myself to come to all the functions. I couldn't make myself visit, Earl I barely ever came to see my dad at Blue Lakes. I regret it now, but I couldn't stand to see him weak and forgetful. When I would come by he wouldn't even know who I was. He was always my hero and that's how I wanted to remember him. Was that terrible?"

"No," I told her. "You did what you had to do. No one can blame you for that. I watch families come and visit all the time; some deal with it differently than others but the one thing they all have in common is that they love the ones they come to see and they all wish it didn't have to be the way it is. Someday there will be a cure. Hopefully, the cure will come sooner than later."

Anna reached out and gave me a small hug. "You're a good man Earl; let's get your tools picked up and loaded into your van so you can get home to that lucky wife of yours."

"That sounds good," I said. I finish up and head out. Once I pull out of her neighborhood and out onto the open road I find myself remembering my own dad. It's a short time we have with those we love, thank God for memories.

Flirty Britches

Every day a man can use a compliment. I'm sure a woman wouldn't mind one every few minutes and I firmly believe that that's what they deserve. A woman is to be admired and listened to; trying to fix or understand the depths of her foundation is about as large of an undertaking as breaking down the complete works of Shakespeare in an afternoon. It can't be done well, if at all. The women at Blue Lakes are a pool of characters, to say the least. Flirty Britches is one of my favorite residents at Blue Lakes; this may not be her real name but it should be. Although she is wheelchair bound, she is more likely to say the darnedest things than not. She is a spark in my day here at Blue Lakes. When I show up in the mornings I have come to look for certain residents before really getting into my work orders or renovation projects. It's like when you were in school and you would show up in the mornings. First, you locate all your friends and then your foes; at that point, you know where you stand in beginning your day.

Flirty Britches gives me a compliment every morning and not just a compliment but also a kiss on my cheek. It is a ritual that she has insisted upon from the first time we met. I don't know if I remind her of someone else or not. From my perspective, it doesn't matter. I want her to be happy, that's all. It's not just me who is the beneficiary of the kisses and quirky comments; I would say most anyone that passes would get a dose of her friendliness. I don't know where she gets her cheerful spirit when to look at her you might feel that life has really handed Flirty Britches a plate of lemons. She has made lemonade out of them from where I stand. Her body seems to be frailer by the day and her motor skills are depleting, yet her spirit is strong.

I must admit that I look forward to her little pick me ups. Confidence in one's self is all fine and good but the human spirit can always use a compliment. She tells me how handsome I am and I make sure to return the favor. I think her flirting keeps her alive. Her son comes to visit her pretty much every other day. He is used to her ways and seems proud of her in spite of all her unfiltered gestures and comments that unfold. They are close; they seem to be untarnished by the rough road of Alzheimer's. I cannot say that about most of our families at Blue Lakes. The loss of memory of their loved ones tends to overshadow the positivity and good times. I think the resident's family members are true warriors. Their visits can be painful; yet not coming for some is not an option. Still, others can only seem to muster up a visit on special occasions. If you really think about it, the ones that visit less frequently might reflect a normal reality. People are busy. Most people have full lives and kids of their own to raise so the occasional visit, if they're anything like me, is more normal than not. The decision to bring someone into our community is a tough one I'm sure. Handing over the care of strangers is unnatural yet necessary; no one wants to have someone else take care of their mom or dad. In their defense, I have heard it said that Alzheimer's is the disease that kills the caretakers first. The effects of dementia and even worse, Alzheimer's is daunting at best. I'm confident that the parent or family member who has been stricken with these terrible circumstances would want the best for their family and would want them to move on with their lives as best as possible. The women at Blue Lakes still have their histories, quirks, and demeanors and thank God for that. They have already had their influence outside of these community walls and now are continuing their journey here. As for the rest of us, we are all just doing the best we can along the way, and I am lucky enough to get a daily kiss on the cheek from Flirty Britches.

26.2

Harry had a fast walker that was custom painted cherry red. It had special pads on the front two legs that were slick and made out of some weird polyurethane. The red walker sported racing stickers from various running events that his son had applied. He also added a small red license plate that had his dad's name Harry printed in big white letters giving the walker a not only a personal touch but doubling as a reminder so his dad would be able to remember that this fine walker was his. Harry came from a running family. His father was a marathon runner in Ireland before coming to America; he then went on to running races all over the United States once he had married Harry's mother and becoming a citizen. Running and walking was clearly still in the blood of Blue Lakes new resident Harry Wood; he had been plagued with early onset Alzheimer's and appeared to be in his late fifties or early sixties. His dementia was certainly debilitating yet he seemed to have maintained his natural urge to run; his speech was a bit muddled yet it was clear that he wanted to stay fit and he wanted to race. I asked his son how long it had been since he had last been truly fit enough to race, and he said it had been years since his dad had the full mental capacity to run in competitions. It was a big psychological blow to Harry because of running being such a tradition in his family. I told his son that we would do everything we could to make his dad's stay with us a good one.

I have watched many of our residents in my time with Blue Lakes walk excessively. It is a common stage of Alzheimer's to go into the Sun-downing phase. This is an exhausting stage for the residents as well as those charged with their caretaking. From what I have seen of our residents, this constant walking and searching seem to be universal among people with advanced dementia. I'm not sure what is going on in the mind of those going through this stage but if I were to try to walk a mile in their shoes with my limited medical knowledge I would say it's a grasp at understanding and desperately trying to get back to some kind of clarity. I can only imagine the inner insanity I would personally feel if I could not string one thought to the next. Searching and moving towards something might not be as different as the quest a toddler might go through in his or her own early development when it comes to trying to figure out what things are and where things are kept. That is just a guess on my part. I know about carpentry and managing a building's upkeep; outside of that, I am just trying to figure out how to help our residents with a bit of dignity and respect. That seems to be the best thing I have found to give them. They may have lost certain motor functions, but no one ever loses their need for dignity.

Getting to know Harry has caused me to pay more attention to the other residents and to notice their walking routines. I like to watch Thelma; she has been with Blue Lakes for about eight months now. She too is a major walker. I'm not saying she could keep up with Harry on her best day, but she is without a doubt the second runner-up in distance walking. I would venture to say that she only sleeps about three hours a day and the rest is spent on searching for new territory within the walls at Blue Lakes. Connie Kintrel is another one of the marathoners living in our community. Another thing I have noticed is that sometimes those who tend to walk a lot have a tendency to pick up followers. It's as if they are suspected of having secret knowledge that some of the others might be missing. For example, Connie has Louise as a follower. I suppose it is just as common as the rest of us to form a kindred spirit with someone; it is uncommon to see Connie without Louise at her side. They travel together, eat at the same table, and watch the same programs in the TV room. There are the two ladies that sit at the entrance to our lobby every single day. We never have to listen for the doorbell because these two ladies make a public announcement each time someone approaches the front door. Friendships are formed throughout the community; I enjoy seeing this kind of normality amongst our residents. It shows that they still are having certain needs met in spite of the obstacles they face.

The days and weeks pass by and I have found myself watching Harry more and more. Each day he walks and trots at a steady pace, only stopping for restroom breaks, a shower, food, and a few hours of sleep when one of our associates direct him to do so. His obsession is different than the others; it appears that Harry is actually trying to recapture the loss of his lifelong hobby. The other residents are doing what is more in line with the traditional excessive stage of walking. This has caused me to wonder if there isn't something more that I might be able to do for Harry. Why can't I give Harry another chance to compete in a marathon?

I think Blue Lakes is ready to hold the first ever event called The Harry Wood Walk-a-Thon. He is doing it already and so is many of our residents. They have been in training for a long time. That's it we're doing it. The first thing I have to do is get permission from Mrs. Whitfield, after that, I will contact all of the family members that are likely to have someone living with us that would be a good match for the walk-a-thon. I have counted about seven residents in all that would be candidates and at least fifteen more that will be glad to walk around and join in the day's fun in a capacity suitable to their own taste. We can have a few associates push the wheelchair-bound residents who cannot push themselves as long as the families are on board, which I'm sure they will love the idea. This will be billed as a fun for all type of event yet I will be sure to have Harry and those participating in the walk set up to walk through a course that will look as real as I can possibly manage. I'm thinking about taping off the designated track on the floors in bright florescent orange tape. There is plenty of room in our community to do this in the hallway that circles around the activities courtyard. The spectators will have full access to the entire course because of its central location. I will encourage the family members to make signs to hold up as the residents around the course like you might see in a real marathon. I believe fifteen laps will be a good distance to set; because of the length the walkers will be going and considering the speed they should be traveling at, this should be a suitable undertaking. I fully expect some of the walkers to venture off course and decide that they would prefer to explore other parts of the community mid-race. Although we will try to keep everyone on course, it is for their enjoyment so the rules will be quite flexible. I can tell you from the excitement of Harry and his family upon hearing about the race; Harry will go the distance. I'm thinking we can have a first place trophy made and enough ribbons for all the residents to receive one at the end of the race.

After three weeks of planning, today is a perfect day to race. The weather is nice outside so I have the residents that are participating outside near the front entrance to the community. I have the front doors propped open for all the racers to enter the community where they will be greeted with cheering and clapping by the staff and family members as they enter the building. The activities department created a great banner that hangs over the starting line that reads, "Welcome to the First Annual Harry Wood Walk-a-thon." Harry was particularly pleased with the banner. We took several photos with many of the residents this morning standing in front of the banner. I wasn't sure how everyone would feel or how tired they might be afterward so I thought getting photos while they were fresh would be advantageous and flattering. I will be snapping off plenty of pictures myself with my phone as the race unfolds. The activities director is a very good photographer and has volunteered her talents. I'm sure there will be plenty of cameras being utilized by family members as well. Orange juice and muffins were passed out to everyone watching and participating to help keep everyone's early morning energy off to a good start, and there were plenty of bottles of water served as well. The activities department was also kind enough to make signs that were pinned to each walker; the signs contained their racing number and their names. We have also designated certain staff members to attend to the residents, so we are sure to keep up with their individual needs. Harry's family arrived early in the morning and helped us with the setup. They were so completely thrilled to be able to Harry back in action after so many years. I counted at least fifteen to twenty family members that showed up for Harry's event. It was impressive. We definitely were going to have our community packed with cheering families today. Mrs. Whitfield waved from across the hallway to me as she entered the building and gave me the two thumbs up for my efforts.

She then mouthed the words, "Great job." I, in turn, mouthed the words, "Thank you," back to her.

What a day this would be. I don't know if the walkers will continue and make the fifteen laps or get side tracked, but in the end, Blue Lakes is celebrating life with its residents and that can only end well.

The racers began to take their positions at the starting line. One of our associates called out for the rest of the racers to take a ready position; she then blew her whistle and the race was on! Harry was purposely placed about ten people deep into the running crowd to give him a better sense of competition as he would surely soon make his way to the front of the pack. Thelma was first off the line grinning ear to ear.

Her granddaughter was visiting from New York City and was yelling with the best traditional accent you've ever heard. "Give it all you got Ma! You're doin' great! You're doin' great!"

Mr. Mascis was blazing his own trail as he was being pushed by one of our associates. It was such a sight to see this young associate encouraging Mr. Mascis yelling out, "I'm racing, I'm racing!" he said, all the while laughing out loud. The associate called out, "We've got this Mr. Mascis, keep going!" Mr. Mascis was laughing, having a great time right off the bat. Mr. Zimmerman was next in line coming down the hallway with all the speed of an Olympic box turtle. It was great watching his face as he walked, you would have though he was breaking new speed records by the look on his face yet he moved at a snail's pace.

I shouted out to him, "You can do it, Mr. Zimmerman, you can do it!"

Mr. Zimmerman stopped to look around for who was calling him. I felt bad for halting such breakneck speed so I jumped onto the course in front of him and motioned for him and the others to walk as fast as they could. I turned and walked the first couple of laps giving encouragement to all the residents that needed it. I looked back to see Harry making his way through the pack. He had the most serious look on his face. He meant business and that was obvious. It took about three laps for him to catch Thelma who was having the time of her life. The families had made signs for their loved ones saying things like, "I love you" "Go fast, Be careful"; my favorite was one that said "Speed Limit 55" and underneath it said, "Go 70!" I took the time to step back and enjoy what was happening. Life can really test a person; I feel lucky to be here and to have been given the freedom to work outside the box. I was hired to be a maintenance man and I must admit I wasn't sure if I was going to make it here after that first day when I had my germ-a-phobic panic attack. I'm so glad I stuck it out. I love these residents as if they were my own family. I guess they are in many ways. They teach me more about life than a lot of my own family members have been able to. I guess you have to be in the right space to learn life's lessons. Today the residents and their families are getting the smiles and excitement they deserve. Good times.

Harry rounds the hallway corner making his way down the stretch that marks another completed lap. He picks up his pace and walks past Thelma and moves into the lead.

They both politely say hello to one another, "Hello, I'm Harry," Harry said, introducing himself to Thelma for what can only be the 100th time. He introduces himself to her every day.

"Hello, I'm racing," Thelma says back to him grinning the whole time.

It was priceless. Connie and Louise were doing quite well until they passed by the activities checkers and bingo room.

Connie stopped and said to Louise, "Are they having bingo in there today?"

Louise answered with great authority, "Yes they are, let's go in and get us a seat."

And so they did; they went into the almost empty room and pulled up a seat and waited for someone to start the game. Sir Richard sat on the couch in the activities room with his walker place right in front of him. He had a serious look on his face and stared forward intently. We tried to get him out earlier but he insisted he would run the race right where he was. I saw no reason to argue with him. He was extremely focused and since none of his family was here today I thought I would let him enjoy the race his own way. I guess we should have shut the door before the race. No worries, the race was still in high gear, I whispered into one of our associate's ears to give them a couple of minutes then get them back in the race if she could. She smiled and said she was on it.

We were at lap fourteen now and it was clear that Harry was well on his way to winning the race; he had already lapped most everyone more than once. Thelma kept her second position and except for two or three associates pushing residents, most everyone else had decided to sit the rest of the race out and were all sitting in the dining room celebrating their own personal victories. You would have thought at least half of them had already won the race by their good moods. What was surprising to see was Mr. Zimmerman was still going strong; his snail pace had picked up about a quarter notch and was powering through the final laps with his family's encouragement. Since the pace was as slow as it was and no one wanted to stay for three more days waiting for everyone to complete the race, we had let the families know that we would consider the race complete once one of the residents hit the fifteen laps. Everyone was on the same page with that idea. I watched Harry for the remaining laps; this was his race and he had kept unbelievable focus; I wondered if he, like most of the others would slowly fade out as the race went along. Harry never showed any signs of forgetting what he was doing; he seemed to be in a place that he remembered so clearly. It's like the examples that I have seen playing certain songs and styles of music for the residents. You can watch their

163

faces transform to clarity when they hear something that takes them back in time. I guess there are sections of the brain that are spared from dementia like perfect time capsules waiting for their cue to open. Racing was Harry's special place that he has been able to store so well that it could not be robbed.

You would have thought he was running a constant seven miles an hour with the breeze blowing across his youthful face. In his mind I imagined there were family members that have long since passed away cheering him on; his dad next to him keeping a slightly faster pace all the while saying to his son, "Come on Harry, racing is in our blood."

I really don't know how many memories he was reliving. I do know by the smile on his face as he crossed the finish line having completed fifteen laps, that this was good for Harry. This was good for everyone involved. Thelma came in second; Mr. Zimmerman was third. After his first lap, something must have clicked because he was able to get his pace picked up to be competitive. I'm thinking he was very proud of himself, as was his family. He ended up being the wild card here today and in my opinion, one of the residents that I would not have thought would finish. Today's race certain seem to have triggered something deep inside of Mr. Zimmerman that none of us at Blue Lakes had seen in him.   That just goes to show that there is much more inside all of our residents that we have yet to discover. Most of the families spent the rest of the afternoon celebrating and visiting with their loved ones.

I stayed long enough to put the community back together so it would be ready for the next day's activities. I had just started pulling up the tape that marked the lanes in the hallways when Mrs. Whitfield was passing by; she suggested I leave it for a few days so the residents could continue the course if they wanted to. I thought about the day's event as we wrapped up the last bit of clean up. Today was a win-win for everyone. Families were able to share new memories and all the residents all had their cups filled in one way or another. I walked out the back door to go to my van, and on the way out I noticed the lake in the backside of the property. The sun was just setting and the air was calm. I decided to walk over and get a better look. There are a small fish jumping up here and there. The sun is reflecting its blue and pink magic hour hues across the water. I wish my wife could see this; she would love it. I remember my first few days at Blue Lakes. I'll never get that image of dancing with the residents and being slimed by the yellow goo. That was the day I panicked and ran over to this same spot. What a difference this past year has made on my life. I've seen so much around here since then. I've seen the hard times on family member's faces as they watch their parents decline, as well as the calm that comes across their countenance as they see their mom or dad enjoying the last chapters of their lives. I feel so blessed to be working here; I look back towards the building and soak up a few more seconds of appreciation for how well today went. As walk over to my van, I wonder to myself if they will remember any of this tomorrow. I hope so.

Hibiscus

This morning I will be confirming water pressure and temperature checks in the number Seven hallway. I've been able to test all six hallways but, as always, I saved hallway seven for last. This is the hallway that houses several of the residents that I have been able to form a bond with in one way or another; there is Mr. Penderson, who I affectionately refer to as Uncle Albert, and Sir Richard. Then there is the room of Mrs. P. I don't know her full name because Mrs. P is the only name in the year and a half that I have been here I have heard her called. I can't say I know her.

Mrs. P has been at Blue Lakes for over ten years now from what I have been told. She lies in bed and looks out her window day after day. Her bedridden state has not changed for several years now; her body is perfectly healthy, especially for her age. Early-onset Alzheimer's has robbed her and her family of the golden years of her life. I never had any interaction with Mrs. P directly, I couldn't say if she heard me when I would come by for my routine room checks or not. She has a faraway stare that involved the memories and a long life that I was not privy to. Out of respect for her and her family, I tried to keep my visits to her room brief and purposeful. There was a timeless quality within that particular room that none of the other rooms possessed. Mrs. P was an institution all her own at Blue Lakes; she had resided there longer than anyone else.

Her room had the feeling of an old comfortable Southern home. Upon entering the front door an obvious transition would come into play. The room was plush and inviting, and you could tell that no expense was spared in all the care and comforts that were available in setting up her room. An old yet perfectly restored pale blue velvet tufted fainting couch was the first piece of furniture that you saw upon entering her room. The tasteful combinations of varied hues of the color blue permeated the entire room, which was also the largest room that was offered at Blue Lakes. Most every room here at Blue Lakes has walls that are painted Baker's Tan with satin white trim; it's a tasteful choice, yet not as obviously elegant as Mrs. P's room.

An oil painting hangs on the wall directly across the room as you walk in the front door. It has a silver colored old wooden frame that surrounds a gray background. The featured image is Mrs. P. The painting shows how beautiful she was; it also captures Mrs. P in an earlier time of her life. Her hair was already silver in the painting, and she had a deep dignified widow's peak that you rarely see these days. The room houses two identical wing back chairs, covered in a silky white material; the legs of these chairs were like no others that I have seen. I studied classical furniture styles a few years back while doing some of my higher end remodels, so seeing all of this in person is a real treat. There was a detailed variety of custom woodworking, shaping and intricate carvings within the furniture that united all the furnishings in the room. An antique game table with four surrounding Queen Anne style chairs was positioned in the far corner of the room. It's clean and has only three items on its glass top, a deck of cards and two magazines; one was Southern Accents, the other, Woman's Wear Daily. Everything in this room had a purpose and a place. No piles of things to get to, just class and a memorialized likeness of an earlier period of Mrs. P's life.

Her daughter has an additional cleaning company that comes in twice a week, once to deep clean and once to freshen the room up. They have done it this way for the past ten years and although our housekeeping department is top notch, they do things the way they want them done. I'm ok with that; our lady contributes a little here and there to accommodate any extra housekeeping needs the might come up from time to time. I get my digital thermometer out and turn on the restroom faucet hot water. After about a minute of running the water, I get my hot water reading. It is supposed to average one hundred and ten to one hundred and fifteen degrees to meet the safety checklist requirements. I'm getting a one hundred and thirteen-degree reading so we are in good shape. It is my habit to troubleshoot the room for any maintenance related problems while I am in the process of temperature checks; it's a good thing I did that this morning because the tank has a small drip of water running down the toilet base when it is flushed. This is a common occurrence after a year or so of use. The rubber gasket that transitions the tank and toilet base wear out from having been leaned on so often, and they will develop a flat spot that allows water to seep out. It's my plan to go ahead and pull the toilet tank and replace all the hardware and gaskets since the inner workings are showing age and deterioration. I fill out my weekly inspection reports while still in the restroom. Mrs. P. is sleeping as far as I can tell so I don't want to disturb her with the additional room checks by turning on the lights or pulling nurse call cords.

Just as I was finishing up my data entries, someone entered the room. I call out maintenance at a low volume so they will not be startled by my presence. It is Mrs. P's daughter and the caretaker that was hired by the family. I was surprised not to see the caretaker in the room when I came in; she is usually here when I come in to do my room checks. In the entire time, I have worked her I have never actually spoken with Mrs. P's daughter. I've heard that she comes on the weekends more often than the weekday, which is most likely why we have not crossed paths. Although I have met and talked to most of the immediate family members, there are a few that I have yet to meet.

"Hello," says Mrs. P's daughter as they come into the living room with a few bags of what looks like groceries and a vase full of flowers.

"Good morning, I was just taking care of the room checks. I found something in the restroom that needs attention. Would it be alright if I took care of it this morning?"

"Oh absolutely, what is the problem?" she asked.

I told her about the leak and said it would take me about an hour to pull the old parts out and replace them with new ones.

"I will need to cut off the water for the maintenance. Are you sure that this will not be an inconvenience? I don't want to get in the way of your visit."

I asked this to make sure it was a good time; I could have easily taken care of this later in the day since the leak was very small and only happened when it was flushed.

"Oh no, it's fine. If you could give us a couple of minutes to put these things away I would appreciate it. Peggy, would you be so kind as to add a little water to the flowers that I brought in for Mom?" She holds the flowers up as she was speaking. "Look at these flowers," she says to me, "Have you ever seen such beautiful gladiolas?"

I say, "No ma'am, I don't believe I have."

She put them on the game table and said to the caretaker as she is coming over to the table with water for the flowers. "Oh Peggy I'll take care of that, thank you. And what is your name?" she says to me.

"My name is Earl Hadley," I say to her with a smile. "Are you Mrs. P's daughter?"

She walks over to and reaches out to shake my hand. "I most certainly am. My name is Ginger, I am so very pleased to meet you, Mr. Hadley."

Ginger is in her mid-fifties as best I can tell. She is well dressed, classic yet not ostentatious. You can see shades of what she looked like in the 50's and 60's, smart hair, never without gloves or a hat. You can see that in some people, it's like that era was just yesterday. We all have certain things that we still cling to. I think Mrs. P's daughter Ginger is very nice and has an abundance of class.

"I'm pleased to meet you as well, Ginger. Let me get the materials together to take care of your mom's bathroom," I say as I walk towards the front door, "I will be back in just a few minutes."

Ginger says from her mom's bedside, "That sounds like a plan Mr. Hadley."

As I walk out the door I can hear her talking to Mrs. P. She tells her about the repairs that are going on in her bathroom and the morning errands. I look back in the room just before leaving to see Mrs. P awake and looking out the window, seemingly oblivious to all of our conversations. I wonder to myself what she is thinking deep down in the still working parts of her mind and memory. Whatever it is it seems to be outside her bedroom window and not at all here at Blue Lakes.

On my way to my storeroom, I walk past Sir Richard who is strolling down the hallway with his walker.

He asks me, "When is the race going to begin?"

I almost laugh out loud but keep it to myself and give him a smile saying, "Sir Richard, the race won't be today, you still have plenty of time to train for it. Did you enjoy the last race we had here at Blue Lakes?"

He looked very proud of himself, confidently exclaiming, "Oh yes, you know, I was the winner, I'm going to win the next one too."

I smiled and said, "That's great, you must be very proud, I remember watching you in the race. You were very fast. Sir Richard I've got to go. I've got some maintenance to tend to. I need to go earn my keep." I was so pleased that Sir Richard remembered the race. I'm glad he thought he won. If that makes him feel encouraged then it's all good. "We can talk about the race again soon, Ok?"

"Alright, you have yourself a good day son," he says with a proud smile.

I wished him a pleasant day and got back on track to gathering materials for the repair. Once I reach the storeroom, I quickly gathered up the needed supplies and head back to Mrs. P's room to get her bathroom leak taken care of. Since I was going to have to pull the tank, I decided to pull the base of the toilet as well to replace the wax ring. This should eliminate all the potential breakdowns or leaks for a long time. I roll my cart to Mrs. P's front door and gently knock on the door.

"Come in," I heard someone say from inside the room.

I opened the door and was greeted by the Mrs. P's caretaker. She is very friendly and welcomes me into the room saying, "Hello, come on in. I hear you're going to repair a water leak for us. "

I reached out to shake her hand and said, "Yes ma'am, I've seen you before but I don't think we've been introduced, my name is Earl Hadley."

"I'm Peggy; it's very nice to meet you. You've been here for over a year now haven't you?"

"I have, close to that, I think it's closer to a year and a half now," I said to her as I watched her putting away the toiletries into the bathroom cabinets.

"They couldn't seem to keep anyone here long term before you came on board. I think we have had over six maintenance men before you came. Well, let me get out of your way."

I tell her she is not in my way and that I've always meant to speak with her but our paths did not conveniently pass. "How long have you been with Mrs. P, if you don't mind me asking?"

"Oh, it's been quite a few years now. I think I've lost track, at least ten years that I know of; I've been friends with Ginger since college. After I retired from nursing at a hospital in Virginia and my husband passed away, Ginger asked me to help out with her mother and I've been a part of the family ever since." I hear Ginger asking Peggy whom she is talking to from the other room.

Peggy says back to her, "I'm speaking to our maintenance man, he was just commenting on how great of a job I have been doing around here, I told him I just enjoy earning my keep," she laughs out loud.

I say to her with a grin, "That's my line; I always say to the residents that I have to earn my keep."

She laughs and tells me, "Oh, I kid with Ginger all the time about earning my keep, she's a hoot. Don't tell her I said so, but you will never meet a finer person in your life. You know I can't remember what you said your name was?"

"This community has that effect on people, there are days that I lose my keys and can't remember where I put them for the life of me. I stay pretty busy though, I'm sure that's why." I tell her she can call me Earl or Mr. Hadley, whichever name she is comfortable with.

"I like Mr. Hadley, that name suits you just fine", she says, "I knew a Hadley when I was growing up as a young girl. Do you have any family down in Baton Rouge?"

"Not that I know of, most of my family comes from around Houston, Texas. I suppose a few of them could have gone to Louisiana over the years."

She goes on to say, "Maybe so, you know Mr. Hadley, all the better people end up in Louisiana!" She laughs out loud again, "Oh I'm just playing. I've got to run out to the drugstore, we forgot a couple of items on our list. It was a pleasure to finally meet you, Mr. Hadley."

I say, "Yes ma'am, it was very nice speaking with you, we will have to do it again sometime."

"Alright Mr. Hadley, If Ginger asks, tell her, oh, let me tell her. Ginger, I'll be right back, I'm running over to the drugstore."

Ginger calls from the extra room, "Ok Peggy, thank you." Peggy smiles at me and goes out the door.

I walk into the bathroom and get started with the toilet rebuild. Once the two tank bolts are off then the job will be smooth sailing. If the bolts have deteriorated too much then I will need to cut them off with a hacksaw blade. I attempt to give the tank bolts a couple of turns and realize that they are both rusted and fused together with the nuts to unbolt. That's fine with me. I've learned a long time ago that you can spend more time being frustrated over what it will take to fix something than to actually fix it. I like being in my forties; maturity is a blessing. I get on my back and start slowly cutting on the tank bolts. Ginger walks into the bathroom and says, "Oh my goodness, we've really put you to work today haven't we?"

I reply, "It's all part of the job, I'm glad to do it. Once I get these two bolts off everything else should be smooth sailing. Getting the old mounting bolts off is always the tricky part."

"Well I'm glad you found the leak, I've heard from some of the associates here at Blue Lakes that you are really good at taking care of the building. I'm glad they have someone like you around here."

"I appreciate that Ginger, it's a great job, I like getting to know the residents; they really have a lot to offer, even in their struggles with dementia and Alzheimer's."

Ginger says to me, "They do indeed."

I ask her how long her mom has been staying at Blue Lakes.

"Oh it's been many years now, I believe she is in her eleventh year here. Mr. Hadley, it seems like she has lived here for a short lifetime. We brought her here about fifteen years after Alzheimer's set in. We had her at home for those first fifteen years before it became obvious that we would need to do something else to accommodate her increasing medical needs. She was quite a handful before we made the decision to come to Blue Lakes. Mom was a real firecracker. It was like watching Dale Earnhardt go around the track in her early days when she used a walker. Oh my goodness, she could go fast. We had slate floors so we had to put tennis balls her walker to slow her down. I was scared to death that she would fall. That made her so mad she could just spit when she realized her walker had the wheels taken off, not that she would actually spit."

"She pushed and tried anyway. She was a determined woman; she still is. Her body is fit as a fiddle for a woman her age. She just doesn't have her full set of faculties anymore. From time to time she will see something that really gets her attention. It only happens every so often, but it happens. We finally moved her here after multiple rides in an ambulance for visits to her doctor. That was the only way she could safely travel. This place seemed like the best option for caring for my mom."

I asked, "What about your father?"

Ginger smiled and said, "My dad was an amazing man, Mr. Hadley, he ran one of the largest commercial construction firms in the state of Louisiana. He was a very accomplished man before he passed away."

I asked Ginger, "How did he die if you don't mind my asking?"

Ginger replied very quietly, "Leukemia, it was awful. Mom's Alzheimer's had set in long before he passed away so he was faced with that as well as his own disease at the end of his life. He hated watching her suffer; he loved her so much."

I said to Ginger, "I bet he did."

"He and Mom had a ritual that they shared every year. Dad would buy Mom two dozen red Hibiscus plants for her birthday. He would plant them just outside the windows of their home so she could see them in her back yard. Oh, my mom loved them so much, Mr. Hadley. It was the best present. He really knew how to make her happy. We had such a hard time after he died. Once my dad passed away we literally went months with the burden of having to tell mom that he had passed away and would no longer be coming home to her in the evenings. She would sit in the kitchen every afternoon waiting for him to come home from work. We would try to wait it out, hoping she would forget, but she would get so upset. Then we would have to remind her that he had died. This went on every day for months. She would relive the news of his passing every day as if it had just happened. I guess after a while the stress of it all was too much and she advanced in her Alzheimer's. She finally forgot to wait for him in the evenings to come home from work. It was terrible to watch her Alzheimer's advance but being able to forget that moment came as a blessing."

I was almost speechless but tried to express my condolences, "I'm so sorry, you and your family really had to be strong for your mom. It takes a special family to get through something like that and you're still taking good care of your mom after these years. I'm sure in her own way, she is still very proud of you."

She replied, "Your very kind Mr. Hadley."

I thanked her and began the last stages of wrapping up the work I was doing on Mrs. P's toilet.

"It looks like you've got it on the run now," she said with a relieved voice. "You're very good at your job, Mr. Hadley."

I thanked her once again and wiped the toilet off with a clean rag. "All that's left is to turn the water back on and check for leaks," I looked at her with a playful serious look. "Here we go," I turned the water back on and checked all the connections. I flushed the toilet to make sure all the new gaskets were seated properly and not leaking. "Success!" I said with confidence.

Ginger was all smiles and said, "Thank you so much, Mr. Hadley, and thank you so much for the conversation. I don't think I've talked about those things for years."

"You're very welcome; it's good to remember where we come from sometimes. Let me get out of your way now, I've got a few more work orders to complete before my day is over. It was very nice talking with you Ginger."

Ginger walks me out to the front door of the room and says, "Don't be a stranger Mr. Hadley, you can stop in and visit with the three of us anytime you want."

"I will, you too Ginger," I say while securing the tools and supplies back on my cart. "Have a great day."

"You too," she replied.

I take my cart and roll down the hall feeling successful and ready to take on the next work order. Across the courtyard I see the activities lady starting up some music for the resident's dance class.

She sees me and calls out to me, "Come on over Earl, we need another dance partner."

I smile and say very politely, "Maybe next time."

She encourages several of the residents to call me over to dance with them.

Various residents call me over in unison, "Hey come dance!" "Good exercise!" "We want you!"

"You come over here and we like to dance!" exclaims one of the lady residents.

I flash back to the dancing that I did on my first day here. I smile, shake my head from side to side, take a deep breath and head over to show them how a real maintenance man dances.

It's Not a Bad Thing

I look into her room to see a body worn and ready. Baby is ready to move on. The disease is working overtime and has begun shutting down all of her body's natural functions. Her chest moves with periodical gasps for air. It is only a matter of hours, days or maybe minutes before Baby's mind forgets to tell her to breathe and she leaves this earth. She has had a full life and she has experienced love and family and life. Her journey most definitely continues and the plastic doll that she has so cherished will go on the shelf soon. Years later, only a handful of people will know how that plastic doll brought such joy during this lady's tough struggle with Alzheimer's. No one will ever truly know what memories and secrets Baby told and shared with that little doll.

Watching Baby take her final breaths was an experience that will never leave me. I was the one to see her take her final breath and depart from her life here on earth. She released her last breath and a true peace came over her face; at that moment a new bloom blossomed in the spirit realm, fresh, no worries, new energy. In retrospect, I did not stay there and watch her for more than a minute but it seemed like a small lifetime. Her ending seemed painless and her transition to the spirit realm was a good one. It's not a bad thing to move on and if we are lucky enough to have shared our life with a friend or a lover then it was a good life. This is what I found myself thinking as Baby left. I felt honored to be a witness. I know her family would have wanted to be here but they had all already said they're goodbyes and since it was so early in the morning they had not yet come back to visit today. It's ok; they had been here every day for the past three days. I could tell they had made their peace with all of this as best as anyone can.

It's early Friday morning; Christmas is just around the corner and though we are in the South and having a mild winter, I'm filled with the holiday spirit; so is the rest of the staff. Last week Mrs. Whitfield passed out unexpected bonus checks so everyone has just a little bit higher skip in their step. Blue Lakes is completely decked out with all the traditional decorations and at least 10 Christmas trees in various community rooms so the residents are reminded of the season they are in. Most all of them are soaking it in and enjoying the lights and colorful décor. Yesterday I gave Harry a Santa's hat that he wore all day long. My shift is just about over for the day, and it's been a long day I must say. I still have one more thing to do before I can go home to Ella and the kids.

On my way into work this morning I did something that I have been contemplating for quite some time. I stopped and bought four red Hibiscus plants with several red blooms on them. I grab a shovel and cart the plants to the backside of the building to access the section of grass just outside of Mrs. P's window. I see that Peggy has hung up a few Christmas lights around the window. It really looks beautiful even though it is still light out. I place the four

Hibiscus plants along the outside of Mrs. P's window just far enough so she will still be able to see them as she looks out.

While digging the holes I am able to see her looking out the window from her bed. She does not seem to react to my presence. I smile at her anyway and keep digging. I can see Peggy and Ginger in the room playing cards at the game table. They both waved at me and continued with their game. There was Christmas music playing inside Mrs. P's room. It was a blast from the past for me to be listening to Bing Crosby sings, It's Beginning to Look A Lot like Christmas. They had the volume up fairly high, most likely for Mrs. P's benefit. I lowered the four plants into their new homes and covered up the roots with the excess dirt. As I watered them in I stepped back to review my efforts and felt good about the way they looked. I hope Mrs. P will remember. Even if she doesn't the flowers will be beautiful for her to look at as she looks out her window every day and thinks of whatever it is she still thinks about.

I pack up my tools and clean up all around her window. I take a look at the plants one more time, I'm so glad that I did that. I think I will be just as blessed as anyone from the effort. They are beautiful. As I walk away I take one more look at Mrs. P inside her room. Her eyes are open more fully than I have ever seen them open before. She sees them! She stares at the Hibiscus plants with excitement and sharpness in her eyes. I can't believe what I'm seeing. I wanted her to enjoy them but I wasn't sure if I would ever really know whether or not if she would actually see them, but she did, she is! I gently tap on the window to get Ginger and Peggy's attention. They look over at me and I point to Mrs. P. They immediately see what I am talking about and rush over next to her side. Ginger looks at the flowers and then Mrs. P, and starts to cry with joyful tears. She reaches over and kisses her mom. Peggy is grinning from ear to ear and waving at me, giving me two thumbs up. Mrs. P looks at the flowers with the most beautiful smile you could ever want to see from her. I decide to leave the three of them with this moment. It is for them. That was my intention. Wow, that is so nice. I wave goodbye and walk off looking back every so often to see that they still have not stopped watching the Hibiscus plants and hugging each other. I can't wait to get home and tell Ella about this.

I never pictured myself in a place like this. Life hands you an unexpected road to take and what direction you will drive can only be individual. I have learned more about the despicable disease called Alzheimer's than I might ever have imagined. Had I not been placed in a memory care center by a classified ad in the newspaper and a small push from my lovely wife, I might not have ever known how truly blessed I was. In the end, I am so thankful for this work that I have been blessed with. To experience a small portion of the lives of our residents has broadened my outlook on life and given me tools to see my own life with a little less anxiety. I plan on staying at Blue Lakes until I feel it's time to move on. It is an honor to work here in spite of the emotional challenges. None of the residents at Blue Lakes asked for Alzheimer's and don't deserve to have people quit on them just because it is difficult. What we do that challenges us makes us better people. I have been able to put all the anxiety that reemerged after receiving my dad's note into a healthier place. It was his decision to do what he did, not mine. I can't bring him back by making my own life suffer. Forgiveness is what I have been able to offer up to his memory. That has taken the burden off my shoulders because, in the end, he would want me to be ok. He raised me to be strong and live out loud. One moment of weakness doesn't discount someone's life.

It does bother me that my stepbrother kept the note from me and that he most likely scratched out the information that my dad tried to pass on to me. It's been fifteen years now and nothing will bring my dad back. Whatever problem he had, he took it with him and I am left as a man with my own choices. I chose to move on and be free of it all. Life is so short anyway; mistakes are a dime a dozen and when we can, we should exercise power over the consequences of those mistakes. Ultimately, what will be will be; love and trust are all we have left that can truly wield any power. This power will not free us of trouble or pain, but it will heal our spirits pretty much every time. Thankfully nothing on earth is permanent. Pain is a battle that does not get the final victory. Lord willing and the creek don't rise, we win in the end and we get to run through the next spiritual plateau free and clean. Our stories are precious and they have power.

The next time you are lucky enough to look into someone's eyes, remember to really see them. They are full of hidden wisdom and humor and lessons. If you are lucky like I am you just might get to share some of it. Yes.

The end.

About the Author

Robert Milstid has been creating literary works for over 30 years. His writing first took form as a playwright, authoring two plays, Just a Phase and I Was a Pig for a Day and Nobody Noticed. Both plays were produced and performed in Houston, Texas. Under the direction of the late Bill Morton, a truly inspirational theatrical writer and director, Mr. Milstid became involved in the theater as an actor as well. He studied at the National Shakespeare Conservatory in New York and was a highly active member of a professional theater, Main Street in Houston Texas for several years. In 1989 he and his wife moved to Hoboken, New Jersey, just across the Hudson River from Manhattan. His one-man show, Diary of a Nonconformist was created, written and rehearsed by Mr. Milstid on the roof of his Hoboken apartment. This performance poetry piece was booked at the now infamous, CBGBs in the East Village. He also went on to perform in several plays while in New York City that included the world premiere of Lanny Hill's original play, "Uncle Alton", as well as becoming an active company member of the 13th Street Repertory Theatre. Mr. Milstid began writing an abundant supply of poetry and free verse performance pieces during his time in the city, performing at the Nuyorican's Poetry Café and various other venues. After his son was born in 1991, he and his wife decided to move to Florida. Shortly after moving to Florida, the couple then had a daughter. After several years of performing in

Orlando, Mr. Milstid hung up his acting hat for the most part and began applying his creative efforts at Nickelodeon Studios as a scenic carpenter and went on to start his own custom carpentry business. In 2005 his marriage of twenty plus years came to an end and he found himself starting from scratch again as a single man. The lonely nights in his small apartment gave way to a renewed need and love for writing again. After the economy took a nosedive in 2009, Mr. Milstid took a position at a Memory Care Center/Assisted living facility as a maintenance technician. After a couple of years of working within the Memory Care environment, Mr. Milstid felt an inspiration to begin writing his book, Transitions, which cameos the lives of those suffering from Alzheimer's disease and the struggles of their families. Mr. Milstid completed his first novel, Transitions in early 2013. His second book, Three Wheels Out was released in 2014. The Consequences of Breathing was recently released, 2017. The second edition of Transitions is now out and a sequel is currently in the works.

Writing is a passion for Robert Milstid and with outlines for three new books underway it doesn't appear to be slowing down. His writing is raw, humble, provocative and unpredictable. His genres are purposefully varied so as to offer new approaches to his art. At forty-nine years old Mr. Milstid still rides his motorcycle as well as his mountain bike and skateboard. He loves time with his four children, his amazing wife, and his Jack Russell. A long life in a short time, this is Robert Milstid.

Dear Readers,

I would love to hear from you after you've had a chance to read Transitions and would greatly appreciate it if you could take a moment and offer your thoughts in a review on Amazon.com. My contact information is also on the first page of the book. Your feedback is always welcome!

www.ingramcontent.com/pod-product-compliance
Lightning Source LLC
Chambersburg PA
CBHW071214240726
48654CB00009B/783